# INTERVIEWING

## A Guide for Health Professionals

# INTERVIEWING

## A Guide for Health Professionals

### FOURTH EDITION

**LEWIS BERNSTEIN, Ph.D.**

Clinical Professor of Psychiatry
Adjunct Professor of Psychology
University of California, San Diego

Professor Emeritus
Department of Psychiatry and Mental Health Sciences
The Medical College of Wisconsin

**ROSALYN S. BERNSTEIN, M.A., A.C.S.W.**

 APPLETON-CENTURY-CROFTS/Norwalk, Connecticut

0-8385-4317-0

Notice: The author(s) and publisher of this volume have taken care that the
information and recommendations contained herein are accurate and
compatible with the standards generally accepted at the time of publication.

Copyright © 1985 by Appleton-Century-Crofts
A Publishing Division of Prentice-Hall, Inc.

85 86 87 88 89 90 / 10 9 8 7 6 5 4 3 2

Prentice-Hall of Australia, Pty. Ltd., Sydney
Prentice-Hall Canada, Inc.
Prentice-Hall Hispanoamericana, S.A., Mexico
Prentice-Hall of India Private Limited, New Delhi
Prentice-Hall International, Inc., London
Prentice-Hall of Japan, Inc., Tokyo
Prentice-Hall of Southeast Asia (Pte.) Ltd., Singapore
Whitehall Books Ltd., Wellington, New Zealand
Editora Prentice-Hall do Brasil Ltda., Rio de Janeiro

**Library of Congress Cataloging in Publication Data**

Bernstein, Lewis.
    Interviewing, a guide for health professionals.

    Includes bibliographies and index.
    1. Medical history taking.  I. Bernstein, Rosalyn S.,
1913–    . II. Title.
RC65.B46    1985        616.07′51        84–28255
ISBN 0–8385–4317–0

Design: Lynn M. Luchetti

PRINTED IN THE UNITED STATES OF AMERICA

# Contents

# Contents

# Preface

This volume is intended primarily for students in schools of medicine and nursing.* Traditionally the therapeutic methods emphasized in their professional education have been almost exclusively the application of physical measures. These measures will, of course, continue to be primary in the treatment of physical illness. However, competence in communication, until recently largely overlooked, is now widely recognized as a significant therapeutic skill for the health professional. All physicians and nurses working with patients use both verbal and nonverbal communication. The quality of this communication can determine the degree to which the overall treatment program will help the patient.

In the past it was hoped that traditional courses in psychiatry and/or psychology would somehow provide students in the health professions with appropriate interviewing skills and sensitivity to the psychologic needs of patients. However, studies indicate that such courses have not always had the desired effect. In one study, graduates of medical schools with an extensive curriculum in traditional behavior science courses were compared with those who had had minimal exposure. Neither group of students had developed any significant skill in establishing helpful relationships with patients or in recognizing and dealing with the emotional aspects of illness.

During the last decades there has been an increasing recognition

---

* It has been brought to our attention that this text had been found useful by students in disciplines other than medicine and nursing: eg, social work, dentistry, guidance counseling, psychiatry, psychology. We realize that, in addressing ourselves to medical and nursing students, we have suggested applications to and used examples only from these fields. We hope that this circumstance will not discourage other students. The principles remain applicable and examples will readily present themselves from daily experience in the other professions.

of emotional components of the disease process and of the fact that these are best treated in the context of a positive relationship between the health professional and the patient. Consistent with this development, we have witnessed major revisions in medical and nursing school curricula, with increasing emphasis on the social and behavioral sciences. Particular attention has been given to interviewing skills as the basis for establishing and maintaining the physician–patient and the nurse–patient relationship.

Clinical skill in dealing with patients' problems of living and dying is more than intuitive sensitivity or tact. This skill can be communicated through teaching programs that enable the physician or nurse to learn to respond in ways that will not only strengthen their relationships with patients, but lead to better treatment outcomes.

The physician–patient and the nurse–patient relationships are part and parcel of good medical care. These relationships affect the outcomes of medical and nursing procedures and contribute to the well-being of the patient. There are important consequences for professional satisfaction, of course, but ultimately patients benefit if they are cared for by persons who derive high professional rewards from their work. It becomes apparent, then, that training in the essentials of interviewing should be included in professional education.

Our plan at the Medical College of Wisconsin for teaching these skills evolved into a program in which small student–tutor groups meet weekly for a four-hour session. During the first hour each student interviews a medical, surgical, or obstetrics-gynecology patient at the bedside. We intentionally exclude students from psychiatric wards to dispel the common notion that only psychiatric patients have emotional problems. In the second hour each student has the opportunity to discuss the interview with the tutor and fellow students. The group then decides which patient presents a problem, the handling of which might become clearer by observing the faculty tutor interview the same patient. The third hour is used for a demonstration interview by the tutor. In the fourth hour the concepts and implications of the material elicited are discussed.

In introducing the student to clinical interviewing by this method, emphasis is on understanding the patient-with-a-disease rather than the disease alone. A patient's illness can then be viewed as significantly affecting his or her life pattern.

As our students were engaged in the clinical experience described, a need for a formalized guide or reference was frequently expressed. This book was undertaken to provide such a guide. Its purpose is to supplement clinical teaching and serve as a source to which the student can turn when questions are raised by personal experience. Primarily we have attempted to provide a point of view that may help the student to understand a patient's behavior. Although interviewing skills are emphasized, these must be considered methods of implementing empathic attitudes. Precedents for a systematic exposition of interviewing were few. Carl Rogers has provided one important model, and many of his ideas are adapted here to the medical setting.

The additions in the third edition—chapters on family interviewing, counseling, and working with minority groups (Chapter 11, Social Distance and Patient Care)—were offered because of changes since the second edition and also because of suggestions from students and colleagues. In this fourth edition, these chapters have been considerably expanded to include recent and relevant research. Additions have also occurred in Chapters 10 (Emotions in Illness and Treatment) and 12 (Death and Dying), both part of this text since its first edition in 1970. The wealth of new material on these two subjects is indicative of increased interest on the part of practitioners. Similarly, a new section in Chapter 11 (Social Distance and Patient Care), Working with the Elderly, reflects an increased concern for this group, the fastest-growing "minority" in our national population.

The heart of this book, however, remains the chapters on interviewing. Yet development of skill in interviewing is never seen as an end in itself; it is viewed as one of the bases for effective treatment. It becomes necessary to teach—and learn—through some formalized structure because for so many students interviewing is a difficult, if not mysterious and somewhat intimidating, area.

Our choice of title, *Interviewing: A Guide for Health Professionals,* continues to reflect a conviction that the material in this volume is relevant not only to the medical and nursing professions individually, but also in an interdisciplinary sense. Although physicians and nurses must work together in patient care, there is little overlap in their professional preparation. It is well known that the relationship between these groups is frequently characterized by mutual suspicion, power struggles, and a breakdown in communication. The patient, in the last analysis, is the loser.

With the proliferation of medical specialties, the question of who has primary responsibility for the patient is often raised. Who is to respond to the patient's concerns between the physician's often hurried visits to the hospital? If the physician and nurse were similarly prepared in communicating with the patient, would the physician feel more secure in sharing the responsibility with the nurse of handling the patient's anxiety? Would the nurse be less likely to evade questions with "Ask your doctor," when a patient expresses concerns? Could the registered nurse, who has given up many duties to ancillary personnel, spend more time at the bedside in the psychologic care of the patient? Would cooperation in this area lead to better understanding and communication between the professions in other areas of patient care? By addressing this book to both professions, it is our hope to contribute in some small way to their improved collaboration.

In company with other writers in these times, we are troubled by a dilemma, imposed by long custom, which we have not been able to resolve. We refer to the use of the masculine pronouns (him, his) when actually the meaning involves women as well as men. We have tried to avoid this trap by endless—and tiresome—repetition of "professional," "interviewer," "counselor," and "patient," or by use of the plural pronouns (they, them). On occasion, this wording became too clumsy and therefore we resorted to conventional usage. It goes without saying that sexism is as abhorrent as racism.

Finally, we would like to express our gratitude to Doreen S. Berne, executive editor at Appleton-Century-Crofts, for her encouragement and valuable suggestions.

**L.B.**
**R.S.B.**

# Acknowledgments

**Aldine Publishing Company** Quotations from: Awareness of Dying, Glaser BG, Strauss AL, 1965

**American Journal of Nursing** Quotations from: Reassurance, Gregg D, 1955, 55

**American Journal of Public Health and the authors** Quotations from: The effects of psychological intervention on recovery from surgery and heart attacks: An analysis of the literature, Mumford E, Schlesinger HJ, Glass GV, 1982, 141; Education and counseling in hospital care, Westermeyer J, 1982, 127

**Bulletin of the American College of Surgeons** Quotations from: Editorial, 1959, 44

**Professor John Hinton, M.D.** Quotations from: Dying, Penguin Books, 1972

**Hospital Physician and the authors** Quotations from: "That crock in 714" may be listening, Deaton JG, September 1967, 56; Winning the patient's confidence in your treatment, Adler LM, Wexler M, April 1969, 86; Winning the hostile patient's cooperation, Wexler M, Adler LM, June, 1969, 78

**Houghton Mifflin Company** Quotations from: Client-Centered Therapy, Rogers CR, 1951

**Journal of the American Medical Association and the authors** Quotations from: Journal of the American Medical Association: Care of the young patient who is dying, Easson WM, 1968, 205; Archives of General Psychiatry: Some psychological reactions to working with the poor, McMahon AW, Shore MF, 1968, 18

**Journal of Family Practice** Quotations from: Dying and death of a family member, Geyman JP, 1983, 125; Selecting patients for brief office counseling, Anstett R, Hipskind M, 1981, 186

**McGraw-Hill Book Company** Quotations from: The Management of the Doctor-Patient Relationship, Blum RH, 1960

**Medical and Health Annual** Quotations from: The teaching nursing home: A new concept, Butler RN, 1983, 183. Copyright © 1982 by Encyclopaedia Britannica, Inc.

**Medical Economics** Quotations from: The economics of doing psychotherapy, Ferber S. Copyright © 1968 by Medical Economics, Inc., a subsidiary of Litton Publications, Inc., Oradell, NJ 07649. Reprinted by permission; Psychiatric referrals: Handle with care! Lebensohn ZM. Copyright © 1967 by Medical Economics, Inc., a subsidiary of Litton Publications, Inc., Oradell, NJ 07649. Reprinted with permission

**Medical Opinion** Quotation from: Updating the Hippocratic oath, Veatch R, April, 1972, 56

**Psychology Today** Quotation from: Psychosomatic syndrome, Holmes T, Masuda M, April, 1972. Copyright © Communications/Research/Machines, Inc.

**Resident and Staff Physician** Quotation from: If I become ill and unable to manage my own affairs, Stead EA Jr, February, 1971, 53

**Ross Laboratories** Quotations from: Feelings and their medical significance: The practitioner and his community, Morgenstern JA, March/April, 1972

**The Laryngoscope** Quotations from: Malpractice—cause and its prevention, Rosenthal RS, 1978, 1

**Western Interstate Commission for Higher Education** Quotations from: Postgraduate psychiatric education of physicians: an overview, Branch CHH. In Eighth Annual Training Session for Psychiatrist-Teachers of Practicing Physicians—1967, Feldman R, Buck DP (eds), 1968

**The Williams & Wilkins Company and the authors** Quotations from: Current Medical Digest: A time for dying, Bean WB, Featherman K, 1970, 37

# INTERVIEWING

## A Guide for Health Professionals

# chapter 1

# The Relationship Between the Health Professional and the Patient

To begin a text on interviewing with a discussion of the professional–patient relationship is an indication of its importance in medical care. In some ways, these relationships have certain elements in common with all relationships. They involve two or more individuals who bring to any particular interaction their idiosyncratic needs and ways of relating, adapting, coping. Each relationship contains the potential for bringing into play the infinite range of emotions—positive, negative, ambivalent. Given the appropriate circumstances, any two people can experience in their interaction with each other mild to intense love, hate, liking, disliking, confidence, fear, satisfaction, frustration, involvement, indifference, dominance, submission—to name only some of the possibilities.

Human relationships present further complications in that each of us is dependent on a complex network of interrelationships. For most people, well-being requires positive relationships with family, friends, colleagues, and a host of others of varying degrees of importance. Even the most independent or the most isolated individual needs at times the services of those who provide no more than creature comforts (eg, shopkeepers) or, on occasions of trouble or illness, the help of professional persons.

Communication, both verbal and nonverbal, is the medium through which relationships begin and develop. The *quality* of communication directly influences the *quality* of the relationship. The most ordinary of greetings: "Good morning. How are you?" can convey a multitude of nuances. Depending on the tone of voice, the facial expression, the body posture, it may be heard as, "I'm really glad to see you and am ready to go on with our business together," or at the other extreme, "I'm really not very interested in your affairs."

Physician–patient and nurse–patient relationships are subject to these same principles. Because of their professional nature, however, there are important distinguishing characteristics. In contrast to social and familial relationships (other than parent–young child) in which a high degree of mutuality is implicit, the primary purpose of professional relationships is the optimal well-being of the patient. The knowledge, skill, and expertise of the doctor or nurse are necessary to the patient, often essential to life itself. Inevitably an inequity arises: the professional is in control; the patient is in some degree dependent. The health professional needs to be aware of this circumstance and its basic implication: concern for the patient's welfare must determine the professional's behavior, words, and actions.

While primary attention, especially in emergencies and acute illness, must be focused on the physical condition, the patient's overall situation—the psychologic and social circumstances, way of living, the resources available in the meeting of crises—require understanding and accurate evaluation.[8] These nonphysiologic factors are known to have a potent effect on health and illness. They are particularly important in planning and carrying out treatment programs. Outcomes often depend on the communication between professional and patient: the professional must make clear to the patient the regimen to be followed and the patient must make clear to the professional any questions and problems in so doing. Ideally, the physician or nurse must be able to establish and maintain the kind of relationship in which the patient feels free to tell the relevant facts. In addition to technical competence, then, the professional should understand and be able to use interpersonal skills in the patient's interest. Self-interest and subjective prejudices, never totally absent in anyone, ought to be at a minimum; the professional ought to be able to function out of respect and concern for even the patient of antithetical background and lifestyle.

The patient has, of course, a significant role in the relationship, and must also practice understanding. Although anxiety and regression may be unavoidable in situations of pain and uncertainty, dependence on the professional ought to be kept within reasonable limits. The physician's authority, when used in a professional manner, should be viewed as appropriate, rather than resented or resisted as arbitrary. Patients ought to be aware that professionals are not magicians. Symptoms too long neglected, the common-sense rules of personal health too consistently ignored, may create situations the doctor cannot mend instantaneously. The patient who seeks help, ideally at an appropriate time (obviously not applicable in emergencies), needs to be able to give as accurate an account as possible of the illness and symptoms. A patient should be ready to cooperate in the treatment by understanding and following medical instructions carefully, and ought to contribute relevant information about life-style and personal habits that will affect treatment and its outcomes.

## A MODEL OF THE PROFESSIONAL–PATIENT RELATIONSHIP

It goes without saying that actual relationships often are very different from the preceding description. The health professional may show no interest in the patient's life-style or reactions to illness. By attitudes and behavior the professional may intimidate the patient or lower self-esteem.[5] The patient, on the other hand, may be too frightened or too embarrassed to give an adequate account of the symptoms, may be uncertain about what to report, or defensive when questioned about etiology. The patient may not follow the prescribed regimen. These less than satisfactory conditions may, to a large degree, be based upon the way in which the relationship and communication have developed.

Models of the professional–patient relationship offer convenient conceptualizations for the study of these relationships as they are practiced or as they might be practiced. An examination of these formalizations offers professionals an opportunity to analyze their own practice.

The interested student will find many such models in the literature. One by Veatch,[15] whose major interest is ethical values in medical practice, is representative and cogent. He discusses four ways of conceptualizing the professional–patient relationship.

First, in the *engineering model,* the physician's self-image is that of a "pure" scientist concerned only with "facts" and therefore free from consideration of values in interactions with patients. The attraction of this point of view may well lie in just this "freedom"—or, perhaps more accurately, noninvolvement—but the limitations of such a stance seem obvious. Even the "purest" scientist must make choices, and choices involve ethical considerations. In the practice of applied sciences like medicine or nursing, the professional must constantly make decisions, inevitably based, consciously or unconsciously, on what is considered valuable or important.

Second, the *priestly model* invests the professional–patient relationship with an almost religious aura in which the patient is expected to view the doctor not only as an expert in a medical specialty, but also as an authority on moral issues. The professional's judgment on such matters as family planning or institutionalization of an aged relative is communicated in as authoritative a manner as are medical diagnoses. This paternalistic view tends to remove participation in decision making from the patient and place it entirely in the hands of the professional. This model is seen as potentially contrary to the individual's freedom of choice and right to self-determination.

In the third, the *collegial model,* the professional and patient become colleagues, "pursuing the common goal of eliminating illness and preserving health" (p. 61).[15] While this model preserves the values of trust and confidence, dignity and respect, Veatch views it as unrealistic in light of frequent differences in ethnic, class, social, and economic values.

He prefers his fourth, the *contractual model:*

Only in the contractual model can there be a true sharing of ethical authority and responsibility. This avoids the moral abdication on the part of the [health professional] inherent in the engineering model, and the moral abdication on the part of the patient in the priestly model. It also avoids the false sense of equality in the collegial model. With the contractual relationship, the [health professional] recognizes that the patient must maintain freedom of control over his own life and destiny when significant choices are to be made. This means relatively greater open discussion of the moral premises hiding in medical decisions, before and as they are made. The contractual model provides assurance to both patient and [professional] that each will retain his moral integrity. Patient control of decision-making is assured without the necessity of insisting that he participate in every trivial decision (p. 61).

We agree with this concept of the professional–patient relationship, which suggests an open and responsible partnership. Idealistic as it may seem, it has been found practicable in even crucial situations—decisions about major surgery, abortion, providing honest information about impending death, etc—given a basic attitude on the part of the professional that reflects respect and concern for the patient.

# FACTORS OPERATING AGAINST GOOD RELATIONSHIPS

## From the Professional's Point of View

Although not inevitably so, frequently the professional's and the patient's interests can be in conflict. Probably doctors and nurses are more often the victims of unrealistic expectations by the lay public than any other group of professionals. " . . . the image of the doctor that has come down to us from Hippocrates, the father of Western medicine, . . . [is that] more than most mortals, [he is expected] to be honest and objective, as well as empathic, trustworthy, gentle and kind" (p. 70).[3] Yet, as they are faced continuously with competing demands, with responsibility for life-and-death decisions, it may be a significant psychologic burden for them to live up to that image at all times.

The criticisms most frequently leveled against them are failure: (1) to give sufficient time, (2) to explain the medical findings in understandable terms, and (3) to show interest and compassion for the sick individual. Doctors might respond, with some justice, that they must constantly balance the needs of any one patient against the demands of their total practice.

For example, consider the problems of Dr. A, a family physician, who is making his usual morning rounds, seeing his hospitalized patients. He had a somewhat late start, because he spent part of the previous night caring for an elderly patient, who had become acutely ill. As he reads the chart of Mrs. B, a woman in her early fifties who has been his patient for only a few months, he sees that yesterday's laboratory report has confirmed his tentative diagnosis of a widespread, probably inoperable malignancy. He has observed the woman's husband in the waiting room and knows that he and the patient herself are waiting to talk to him. There are still several others to see in the hospital before he leaves for his office, where, he is aware, the waiting room is already filling up. He realizes that he cannot simply state so crucial a diagnosis to his patient and her husband and then leave. He will have to explain the further medical implications, answer their questions, offer emotional support in the face of devastating news, demonstrate there and then that he will continue to give as good care as possible to Mrs. B—and he is more than usually pressed for time! If he avoids an immediate interview, he runs the risk of his patient learning her diagnosis from other sources, probably less prepared to handle so delicate a situation. If he gives the diagnosis quickly and offers a later appointment for full discussion, he leaves the sick woman and her husband to "stew" in their anxieties and, in the process, almost certainly build up anger and resentment toward him.

To the apparent solution that this doctor must reduce his patient load, another dilemma presents itself. Dr. A is in his late thirties. Just a few years ago, he was still a student, accumulating debts while he completed his training. It is understandable that he allows his practice to grow beyond comfortable limits, wanting the professional and material rewards for which he has waited so long.

He has other conflicts of a similar nature. It goes without saying that his primary commitment is to his patients' well-being, but is the path to that well-being always quite clear? At times, for example, the patient's immediate and long-range interests may be in conflict: eg, Mr. D has a severe skin rash, which is causing him extreme discomfort. The etiology is obscure and the diagnosis difficult. It would be easy to relieve Mr. D's distress by medication and salves. However, this procedure might mask symptoms, further delaying diagnosis and effective treatment.

In other circumstances, while it is generally agreed that physicians must not mislead their patients about their diagnoses and prognoses, in the face of "bad" news, where no medical treatment will accomplish anything more than relief of pain, is it always "dishonest" to use palliative methods, allowing temporary "false" hope in the hopelessly ill patient? To cite another dilemma: the relationship between physician and patient is expected to be almost sacredly confidential, but what is the doctor's responsibility if a teenager "confesses" drug use or sexual promiscuity?

Nurses must cope with similar problems. Nurses may seem more accessible than busy physicians and therefore be questioned with less hesitation. They may find themselves under some constraint, however, if they are uncertain about the information the patient already has or if the requested information is of an unfavorable nature.

But the most serious block for professionals in relating to patients is the gap created when profound differences in educational, social, and economic circumstances exist between them and they cannot talk to each other with clarity or confidence. Professionals and patients may even take diverse views of illness itself. For one, it is a problem in diagnosis and treatment, which professionals can view dispassionately and handle empirically. Training in the scientific method has taught them just this way of trial-and-error problem solving. For the patient, illness is at best a discomfort and interruption of life. At worst, it is a threat to that life, which can hardly be viewed with calm or objectivity.

## From the Patient's Point of View

Except in the unusual circumstances of similarity in training and background, the patient may have difficulty in understanding the illness and the delay or absence of cure. If discussion with the professional is hurried or unintelligible, the patient's anxieties and anger may well interfere with the treatment regimen.

From the point of view of the patient, then, the most serious barriers to a good relationship (and consequently better diagnosis and treatment) are the professional's lack of time, seeming lack of concern, and failure to tell the patient what the patient needs to know and can understand about the illness. Repeatedly in studies and surveys[14] when patients are asked their opinions about medical care, they respond critically and often bitterly about the doctor's or nurse's hurry when taking care of them or talking to them. This "hurry" is apt to be interpreted—and resented—not as a lack of time, but as a lack of humane interest in the sick individual. Failure to discuss the illness and treatment in understandable terms is viewed, not as a difficult problem in communication for the professional, but as a further rejection, intentional or not, of the patient.

## EVIDENCE OF DISSATISFACTION WITH THE RELATIONSHIP

In this inevitably unequal relationship, patients do find means of expressing their disappointment with medical care, often in negative ways that in the long run are to no one's advantage.

They may break off contact with one physician and seek out another, in which case the loss of time and perhaps change in treatment direction may have more or less serious consequences.

## Resort to Quackery and/or Unorthodox Treatment

Of more concern are the number of sick persons who turn to some form of quackery, ranging from harmless but useless measures (eg, copper bracelets for arthritics) to "treatment" that actually harms the patient (eg, removing patients from prescribed medication and substituting unproven, questionable injections, pills, etc, in diagnosed illness such as cancer).

In various studies of the resort to quackery, one finding is well-nigh universal: by giving time and sympathetic attention, sometimes at high fees, the quack offers a sense of caring and inspires a feeling of hope, probably false but nevertheless longed for. The quack thus meets a profound need, which the professionals, rightfully restricted by ethical standards, find it difficult to offer. Fortunately, this restriction need not limit professionals to a dismal either (false hope)/or (no hope) choice. If they understand the fear and desperation experienced by patients, particularly those who face life-threatening disease, they can find ways to make the time to demonstrate concern and compassion, to listen empathically, and to explain, if need be, repetitively.

Unorthodox treatment, which also has a growing appeal for many patients, differs from quackery in that it is seldom unethical or harmful. However, its methods are considered unproven and therefore not recognized by accepted medical practice, even though sometimes used by licensed physicians. These methods range from diet therapy and use of megavitamins to mental imagery and faith healing.

In a study by researchers at the University of Pennsylvania Cancer Center,[4] one surprising finding was that many patients who sought alternatives to conventional treatment were not stereotypical of poorly educated, desperate individuals. Almost 80 percent of the 356 patients interviewed had had some college education and some continued to have conventional care from doctors who knew of, but did not interfere with, the other treatment. Other findings indicated that the quality of the relationship with the doctor influences patients who seek unorthodox care; ie, the poorer the relationship, the more likely is the patient to resort to nonconventional treatment. Further, the researchers concluded that the aspects of the nonconventional that patients wanted could be part of orthodox care—and patients want primarily a caring, ongoing, dependable relationship with their physicians.

Health professionals who are really persuaded of this point of view have taken a long step in the direction of enlightened self-interest. We hasten to add that we are not suggesting self-interest as the only motivation. Yet the conclusion is inescapable that the physician who handles the relationship successfully is less likely to have problems with loss of patients, fee collections, and malpractice suits.

## Nonpayment of Bills

There is considerable evidence that patients who are treated with respect and understanding do pay their bills. On the other hand, many patients who are dissatisfied with their medical care, whether the deficiency is real or fancied, are more likely to use nonpayment to indicate their dissatisfaction. Parenthetically, there also appears to be a definite connection between the seriousness of an illness and nonpayment, perhaps because in a serious illness there are more reasons for the patient to feel threatened and to project this threat onto the physician. This attitude was well illustrated in an interview with a patient who had terminal cancer. The interview was conducted by the senior author before a small group of medical students. The patient told of a radical mastectomy several years prior to her present hospitalization. Immediately following surgery her surgeon told her, "This is as far as I go." The patient inquired whether she need not visit his office and was told there was nothing else the surgeon could do. In the interview the patient turned to the medical students and said, "I hope you won't treat your patients like that. I wanted to see him because I was scared. I needed to talk to my doctor. But he abandoned me. I was so mad, I've never paid his bill. I had a feeling he knew then that the cancer would spread to other parts of my body, and he was scared too—afraid to have me for his patient when it happened. Well, he has the nerve to phone me in the hospital, now that I'm sure I'm dying, and ask about his bill. Well, you can be sure I'll never pay it."

In the above incident we have only the patient's version of what happened, and, from a certain standpoint, there may have been no need for her surgeon to see her further. In rejecting the patient's request for follow-up consultation, the surgeon may even have been motivated by humanitarian considerations—preventing the expense of unnecessary visits. However, he failed to sense that in requesting further visits the patient was communicating her need for understanding and compassion. By his rejection he failed to give recognition to this patient's profound anxiety. He may indeed have been correct in concluding that she was no longer an appropriate patient for him. However, had he been more sensitive to her fear, he might have explained honestly his reasons for wishing to discontinue his care and perhaps worked out a referral, which might have eased her panic in facing her problem alone.

## Malpractice Suits

The literature indicates that suits are increasing alarmingly. Awards to patients have exceeded a million dollars in a single suit. Consequently, premiums for malpractice insurance continue to skyrocket. Even physicians who have never been sued fear the risk of practicing without insurance.

The reasons for malpractice suits have been analyzed in a series of studies conducted by Blum[1] for the California Medical Association. His findings indicate that a breakdown in the physician–patient relationship may indeed be a major cause of malpractice suits. Blum conducted a careful psychologic analysis of suit-prone patients and suit-prone physicians. He used the term *suit-prone* to designate physicians who had been sued and patients who had sued more than once.

The suit-prone patient was characterized as "dependent, emotionally immature, extreme, rigid and authoritarian, incapable of accepting adult responsibility, and quick to suspect and to blame others for his frequent troubles" (p. 105).[1] Many of these characteristics are manifested in patients' wishes that the physician protect and deliver them from all illness. These patients apparently cannot accept the realistic limitations of medical science. They suffer extreme anxiety over matters that others would overlook—a penicillin rash or mild side effects from medication. Other disappointments are more serious but are not always under the health professional's control—death of a family member, a stillbirth. In such circumstances the suit-prone patient finds it easy to decide that the doctor or nurse has been guilty of malpractice.

The possibility of a lawsuit is, of course, increased when a suit-prone patient is treated by a suit-prone physician. The suit-prone physician

> . . . wants patients to look up to him and put their hopes in him. The doctor tries to promise the patients what they want; he fears to admit to them or to himself his own inabilities or inadequacy. He does not warn patients of things that can go wrong nor does he explain the problems in medical care to the patient. He tries to do things he is not equipped to do, and he finds it hard to turn to his colleagues for the assistance they could and should provide in the care of his patients (p. 138).[7]

When confronted with patient dissatisfaction, the suit-prone physician, rather than helping patients feel less angry through discussion and explanation, may dismiss or neglect them. In the studies conducted by Blum, suit-prone patients indicate that their physicians did not discuss their complaints. Furthermore, these patients report that in no instance did the physician admit he may have been wrong. "The physician, by protecting his shaky self-esteem, by not sympathizing with the injured or disappointed patient, or by not admitting error, puts his neck into the lawsuit noose" (p. 139).[7]

The fact that such lawsuits result as much from a breakdown in the relationship as from actual malpractice is further emphasized by interviews with malpractice lawyers. These lawyers report that they had recommended or started action in less than 50 percent of the cases brought to them, primarily because they felt many of the cases had no merit.

If a case should reach court, the personality of the suit-prone physician can further complicate matters. "The physician who acts in an insulting, aloof, or angry manner may well turn the jury against him, as may the doctor who talks down to the jury, casts apersions on his patient, or speaks in confusing medical jargon" (p. 140).[7]

More than a decade after Blum's studies, a Senate subcommittee concerned with hospital costs reported findings very similar to his: malpractice suits and the amount of judgments were continuing to increase sharply. The corresponding rise in the cost of malpractice insurance was reaching levels almost prohibitive for many physicians. Significant was the statement of the causative factor:

> Most malpractice suits are the direct result of injuries sustained by patients during medical treatment or surgery. The majority have proved justifiable. *The suits are the indirect result of a deterioration of the traditional physician–patient relationship* (pp. 55–56).[12] [Italics added]

In a paper presented at a staff conference at the Washington University School of Medicine, Rosenthal,[11] legal counsel to several medical institutions in St. Louis and often called on to give seminars in medical malpractice, writes:

> The physician–patient relationship is thus probably the single most important factor in preventing malpractice claims. . . .
>
> Effort should be made to make the patient feel like a respected and important person, particularly within the hospital setting. This requires the interest and concern of nurses, technicians and orderlies. The patient should be informed of the identity of his treating physician. The treating physician should take primary responsibility for the patient's care and should inform the patient that he is the one to look to for patient problems. The treating physician should tell the patient about the other persons at the institution who will be asking him questions or examining him or treating him. For instance, the patient should be told about the intern and resident who will be responsible for him, the nature of their responsibilities, and what their purpose is. The patient should be informed of all specialists who are called in and the reason

for their presence. If the primary care of the patient is to be provided by anyone other than the admitting physician, this should be explained to the patient. The patient should not be made to feel abandoned within the institution. If the physician who has been providing the primary care for the patient is going to be away from the hospital for any length of time, the patient should be informed. The patient should be told who is to be responsible for his care in the absence of his treating physician and he should be assured that the substitute physician is competent and that he has been fully apprised of the patient's particular problems (pp. 5–6).

A vicious cycle can be set in motion. Poor professional–patient relationships are the basis for many malpractice suits. In turn, malpractice claims and awards tend to encourage physicians to practice, not improved relationships, but a kind of defensive medicine. A 1969 survey by the New Jersey Chapter of the American College of Surgeons[13] leaves little doubt that the professional liability claims have altered methods of practice. Some 66 percent of the physicians surveyed indicated increased caution in discussing diagnosis, treatment, and prognosis with patients and families. An even higher percentage avoid any discussion of another physician's treatment of a patient. Some 60 percent answered "yes" to the question, "Do you find yourself ordering more x-ray and laboratory tests than are really necessary just to protect yourself from malpractice claims?" Further, 61 percent indicated that they were requesting more consultations in an effort to protect themselves from possible malpractice suits.

A survey in 1984 by the American Medical Association[16] indicates that defensive medicine continues to grow. Two in five physicians reported ordering even more diagnostic tests than they did five years earlier. Almost half of those surveyed have increased their referrals to other physicians. In addition, it was found that physicians are reacting to higher liability risks by maintaining more detailed records, refusing certain types of cases, spending more time with patients, performing additional treatment procedures, and increasing fees. This 1984 survey estimates that the annual cost for defensive medicine has grown to over 15 billion dollars, more than the total of malpractice judgments against physicians in the previous year. Not all of these precautions are necessarily bad practice, but the fact is that the increased caution, number of tests, and consultations are often not in the interest of the patient, but for the protection of the doctor. As Rosenthal states:

Malpractice lawsuits are not prevented solely by practicing "defensive medicine." Positive steps can be taken by the physician with the investment of very little time or resources. . . . Time must be taken to discuss the patient's problems and answer his questions in order to help take some of the mystery out of his aches and pains. Before any treatment is rendered, the physician must make sure that the patient understands the risks associated with the treatment and what alternatives are available . . . (p. 10).

Repeatedly, as the problems in medical practice are explored in studies and surveys, seminars, and faculty committees, the need for improved relationships between professional and patient is emphasized. The development of family practice is seen as one effort to achieve this improvement.

## DEVELOPMENT OF THE FAMILY PRACTICE SPECIALTY

The president of the American Academy of General Practice described this new specialty as ". . . built on the solid foundation of general practice but [it] takes off from there into important areas of behavioral science and the vital but little understood health factors in environment and interpersonal relationships" (p. 35).[9]

The specialty of family practice was approved by the Advisory Board for Medical Specialties and the Council on Medical Education of the American Medical Association in 1969 and has since had enthusiastic support and rapid growth. Understandably its beginnings have been controversial, in part because some of its teaching material comes from disciplines other than medicine (eg, psychology, sociology). In the main, of course, family medicine derives from clinical medicine. Primary emphasis must continue to be on the traditional components of clinical training—anatomy, physiology, organ systems, disease entities, etc. However, the point of view has been persuasive that inclusion of relevant education in the social sciences contributes in important ways to effective practice. In the time since it has been an approved specialty, all Canadian and virtually all U.S. medical schools have established departments of family practice. Also, there are numerous opportunities for residencies, increasingly popular with medical students, in community hospitals, clinics, and private practitioners' offices.

The rationale for the development of family practice has been twofold. First, it recognizes that ever-increasing specialization in medicine gives rise to fragmented and depersonalized care. If the family physician has a good continuing contact with all members of the family, the implications for improved and coordinated treatment are clear. The family doctor is also in a strategic position to perform another major function, that of teacher ("doctor" originally meant "teacher"), certainly as important as the role of healer. A family physician can encourage health practices and life-styles that prevent disease and help people to assume more responsibility for their own well-being with less rather than more medical care.

The second most compelling reason for a specialty in family practice is that no other single factor has greater impact on growth and development, health and illness, than the family itself.[6] Whether viewed from the perspective of nature (inherited qualities) or nurture (environmentally determined characteristis) or, more accurately, the combined influence of both, no individual, sick or well, can be understood without reference to family and upbringing. Further, most individuals live in family situations, and one's living circumstances obviously affect health and illness. Any effective treatment program, particularly in prolonged or chronic illness, will benefit from the support and cooperation of those in the immediate environment of the sick person.

The difference between the practitioner who deals with the individual alone and the family doctor lies not in clinical knowledge and skill, which both require, but in the latter's advantage in knowing specific families as families. Optimally, the family doctor's special training will have included theoretical information about family interaction and dynamics. A family physician will have studied in a practice residency or other supervised situation how to observe behavior, and will have participated in interactions with families. Such a physician will not "medicalize"[2] the family, but use what opportunities present themselves to take note of relationships and characteristic ways of reacting to each other and to events. It is recommended by some family specialists (eg, Rakel[10]) that early in association with the family, the doctor, after appropriate explanation, should arrange a meeting at which all members who are living together will be present. There is advantage in holding this meeting in the home in the probable increased relaxation and comfort of the family in familiar surroundings. The doctor will make clear his or her function and responsibility for primary care; will explain under what circumstances he or she use referral and consultation while remaining in charge of overall care; will encourage all members to ask questions and express their point of view, and will help them understand what problems they can safely handle themselves and which will require his or her attention. Consider how far ahead this family physician will be when an emergency or serious illness occurs!

## A Case Example

The following brief example is intended to demonstrate how the family physician's knowledge of a particular family can help in treating one of its members.

Dr. S has known the T family as patients since they came about ten years ago to live in M, the large midwestern city where he practices as an internist and family doctor. The family consists of Mr. T, 49, owner in partnership with his brother of a successful men's clothing store; Mrs. T, 46, homemaker; Thomas, 21, senior at the local university, living at home and working part-time in the family business; Dorothy, 19, sophomore at the same university, living in an apartment with other students and working part-time in a department store; Edward, 17, freshman at an eastern university to which he has earned a scholarship.

Dr. S has treated the children as well as the parents and has been familiar with their circumstances and activities for the past ten years. To his knowledge, there have been no major crises or life-threatening illnesses in the family. He has been aware that Mrs. T, usually self-possessed and cheerful, can become overly anxious and exert considerable pressure on him when the children are sick. At these times, she calls his office several times a day, is concerned that the children are missing important educational or social opportunities, and presses him for additional medication or measures to get them well more quickly. He has concluded that Mrs. T is highly devoted to her family and perhaps overly ambitious and possessive of her children, but had not actually discussed her attitudes with her until a year ago. At that time, Mrs. T had come to his office with complaints of abdominal pain, nausea, and vomiting over a period of two weeks. The office examination proved negative, as did the laboratory tests. When Mrs. T came to his office for a follow-up visit, she reported some improvement, but was still pale and subdued. To a casual inquiry about the family, she burst into tears and sobbingly revealed that she was "losing" Dorothy. It developed that, after several months at the university, Dorothy wished to live with new friends in an apartment. She had resented her mother's opposition to attending an out-of-town university and saw this move as a reasonable compromise. Mrs. T had reluctantly agreed; her physical symptoms began soon after. With a little encouragement, she discussed in some detail her fears of the "breakup" of the family. Dr. S did little more in this visit than listen empathically and tentatively suggest, when Mrs. T at the end of the interview commented that perhaps she was "exaggerating," that it might be time for her to look about for new interests.

His next contact with the family occurred ten months later, when

Edward came to his office for a physical as part of his application to a prestigious eastern university. He could not conceal his pride in having won a scholarship there. As he chatted with the boy, Dr. S inquired about the family. Edward's face clouded and he replied that everyone was fine, "except Mom, who has a bad rash on her arms and face and cries a lot."

When Mrs. T appeared at his office about a month later with the same rash, she explained that she had felt "hopeless" about seeing him sooner, realizing that her present symptoms were "like my problem when Dorothy left and I didn't think you could do anything."

On this occasion, after the examination Dr. S instituted some measures of symptom relief immediately. He also complimented Mrs. T on her recognition that her physical complaints were related to her sense of loss when her children left home. He asked about her reaction to his earlier suggestion that she find a new interest. She admitted that she had not given it much thought, and was not sure how to begin, but felt it might be worth more consideration. He suggested calls to the continuing education department of the local university with a program for older women, and a vocational counseling center.

Over the next several months, Mrs. T visited the office about every two or three weeks for continued treatment of her skin condition, which improved slowly with occasional minor setbacks. For some time, she did not refer to the doctor's suggestion of finding new interests, and he refrained from questioning her. She always spoke at some length about the children's activities, indicating pride in their achievements and some satisfaction in the fact that Thomas was still at home, that Dorothy visited often, and that Edward would be home for his holidays. About four months after her first visit for the skin condition, she announced that this would probably be her last visit for this particular complaint. Dr. S agreed, since the rash was practically healed. Mrs. T added, with a smile: "And I haven't forgotten your other suggestions, Doctor." She explained that, after many discussions with her husband and children, they had all agreed that she would be best satisfied and feel that she was making a continued contribution to the family if she did part-time office work in their store. She had already had an appointment at the vocational counseling center and was planning to follow through on their suggestion that she take a brush-up business course. She had done office work some years before and still had some skills.

One might comment on the outcome in this case that Dr. S was wise to avoid putting pressure on Mrs. T to act on his suggestion, to allow her to arrive at her own decision in her own time, and to continue to treat her with respect and empathy. He had the advantage, of course, of having known her and her family for some years.

One might speculate about the treatment Mrs. T would have had if she had gone first to an internist or dematologist who did not know her or her family situation, or one who practiced "scientifically" with regard only for physiologic "facts." She would probably have undergone innumerable tests. There might well have been several referrals to specialists. Many different treatment procedures might have been tried and, in the end, a psychiatric referral might reasonably have been suggested. Her skin problem would probably have required a much longer treatment period and undoubtedly would have involved far greater expense to reach a satisfactory resolution.

In concluding this discussion of family medicine, it should be pointed out that the principles that underlie its practice are not exclusive to this specialty. Its basic concepts of viewing the individual's health problems in the context of the family and social situation, of taking into account attitudes and life-style in the diagnostic process and treatment plan, are applicable in all fields of medicine and can be used by any practitioner.


## SUMMARY

A positive professional–patient relationship is recognized as essential to sound medical practice and the optimal well-being of the patient. Mutual trust and respect are basic characteristics of this relationship. The interview is the medium for the development of the professional relationship. Therefore medical and nursing education should include specific training in interviewing skills and, concomitantly, an understanding of psychologic reactions to illness and treatment.

A model of medical practice is presented as a concise conceptualization that can be used to study medical care as it is or might be practiced. No one model can be used in all practice or with all patients. The favored conceptualization is the *contractual model,* in which professional and patient respect each other's roles and share responsibility for treatment programs with relative equality.

Factors that operate against good relationships are presented from the professional's point of view and the patient's. The professional, often expected to live up to an unrealistic ideal, usually works under pressure and must constantly make difficult choices affecting the well-being of the patient. Professional and patient may view illness and medical care in quite different terms because of profound differences in background and training. It becomes the professional's responsibility to overcome these differences and make as clear as possible to the patient the nature of the illness and the prescribed regimen.

From the patient's point of view, the problem in relating to the professional is threefold: the professional never seems to have enough time, the professional uses language regarding diagnosis and treatment that the patient has difficulty in understanding, and often the patient misses a sense of caring on the part of the professional.

The evidence that dissatisfaction is widespread lies in frequent change in doctors, patients' turning to quackery and/or unorthodox treatment, nonpayment of medical bills, and ever-increasing malpractice suits. Concern about malpractice suits leads physicians to practice "defensive" medicine—ie, using extensive laboratory tests and consultations—thereby causing considerable increase in medical costs.

The development of the family practice specialty is seen as one effort to deal with the dissatisfactions caused by depersonalized and fragmented medicine. In addition to expertise in clinical medicine, the family practitioner has training in family dynamics and psychologic aspects of health and illness. As the primary care physician for all members of the family over time, the family doctor is in a position to "teach" good health practices and to know what events and interactions are related to health and illness.

In conclusion, we are aware that the import of this chapter may be interpreted to mean that additional responsibilities are placed on the already burdened physician and nurse. We believe that such a conclusion would be incorrect. In succeeding chapters we hope to show that skilled use of relationships not only saves professional time but provides intangible rewards important to physicians and nurses, as well as patients.

# REFERENCES

1. Blum RH: The Management of the Doctor–Patient Relationship. New York, McGraw-Hill, 1960
2. Carmichael LP: Relational model, family, ethics. Presented at the Annual Meeting of the Society of Teachers of Family Medicine, San Diego, May 6–9, 1978
3. Cassell EJ: The therapeutic relationship. In Medical and Health Annual. Chicago, Encyclopaedia Britannica, 1978
4. Cassileth BR, Lusk EJ, Strouse TB, Bodenheimer BJ: Contemporary unorthodox treatments in cancer medicine. Ann Intern Med 101:105, 1984
5. Chafetz ME: No patient deserves to be patronized. Med Insight 2:68, 1970
6. Doherty WJ, Baird MA: Family Therapy and Family Medicine. New York, Guilford Press, 1983
7. Editorial: Breakdown in doctor–patient relationship is shown by malprac-

tice suits, say psychologists in C.M.A. study. Bull Am Coll Surg 44:137, 1959

8. McWhinney IR: An Introduction to Family Medicine. New York, Oxford Univ Press, 1981
9. Michaelson M: Family doctor, space-age style. Today's Health 47:35, 1969
10. Rakel RE: Principles of Family Medicine. Philadelphia, Saunders, 1977
11. Rosenthal RS: Malpractice: cause and its prevention. Laryngoscope 88:1, 1978
12. Schroeder OC: Medical malpractice: old wine in new casks. Postgrad Med 51:55, 1972
13. Thurlow RM: Malpractice: a growing threat to doctor–patient relations. Med Econom 46:212, 1969
14. Tuckett D: Doctors and patients. In Tuckett D: An Introduction to Medical Sociology. London, Tavistock Publications, 1976
15. Veatch R: Updating the Hippocratic oath. Med Opinion 8:56, 1972
16. What's Ahead. Med Econom 61:184, 1984

# chapter 2

# An Overview of Interviewing Techniques

In the first chapter, one of our purposes was to distinguish between professional and personal relationships and to indicate the importance of the professional relationship in medical diagnosis and treatment. In this chapter, as we turn to an examination of the interview itself, we begin by making a similar distinction: between professional and personal conversations, the professional conversation being, of course, the interview.

The nature of personal conversations will vary in relation to a wide variety of factors. Some of these might be the degree of intimacy of the participants (eg, parents discussing plans for a child in contrast to two strangers chatting at a large party), the number of individuals involved, their immediate circumstances, their interests and background. Different as these hypothetical conversations might be, there are two elements that they are likely to have in common. First, a certain mutuality or free give-and-take will characterize most of them, and second, these interchanges among relatives, friends, and acquaintances probably will not have any conscious structure or preconceived purpose.

In contrast, the professional conversation, the interview, takes place under circumstances that implicitly impose certain disciplines. It is held, to begin with, more in the interest of one rather than both of the participants, ie, the patient. It has a definite purpose which in the most general terms is to further the patient's well-being by offering appropriate help in problem-solving efforts. The interview is also usually subject to formalities of time and place: it occurs at a given date and hour, most often in the professional's office. The content of discussions between professional and patient will have as much variety as personal conversations, but always the interview will center around the needs, the problems, and the feelings of the patient.

## PRINCIPLES OF INTERVIEWING

Further, the nature and purpose of interviewing impose certain principles upon the professional. As professionals become aware, during training, of their own verbal and nonverbal patterns, their usual conversational habits must be replaced by more disciplined communication. They must assume responsibility for the conduct of the interview, but avoid the kind of control or rigidity that will inhibit or intimidate patients and limit the patients' verbalizations regarding the problem. Professionals should keep the content of the interview in focus while maintaining flexibility so that relevant material is not inadvertently excluded. They need to remain sensitive to patients' feelings expressed both verbally and nonverbally, so that they can understand the relation of these feelings to the problems under discussion. Their own subjective, personal feelings cannot be permitted expression in the professional situation. They must remain open and accepting toward patients, sometimes even under the trying conditions of hostile, uncooperative behavior.

## CLASSIFICATION OF RESPONSES

The above list of "dos" and "don'ts" may well seem to suggest that the professional is expected to adopt an almost impossible stance, demanding an unusual degree of self-control and an unchanging, constant attitude of concern and acceptance toward patients. It is the thesis of this text, however, that achieving skill in interviewing is neither impossible nor a mysterious, inexplicable gift of a fortunate few, too intangible and elusive to learn or to teach in any practical way. Systematic analyses of interactions in interviews demonstrate that responses can be classified and studied for the purpose of developing proficiency. These analyses have demonstrated that virtually every response falls into one of five basic categories: (1) evaluative, (2) hostile, (3) reassuring, (4) probing, or (5) understanding.[1,5] Any extended interaction such as an interview may, of course, bring several or all of these responses into play.

Below we shall define these five categories and illustrate each as a different way of responding to the same comment from a patient. Following this overview, succeeding chapters will discuss each category in detail, with illustrations from actual medical interviews.

A student nurse is at the bedside of a patient in a veterans' hospital. During the course of the conversation, the patient excitedly exclaims: "I tell you I hate that doctor of mine. I hate him! I hate him! I ask him what's wrong with me and he gives me the brush-off. Tells me a diagnosis hasn't been made yet. I don't believe him! It makes me feel so terrible, especially when I have to count on him to get well. I—it worries me."

## The Evaluative Response

Had the nursing student given an evaluative response, she might have responded to this patient more or less as follows:

"You certainly must get this straightened out. There's no sense in hating your doctor. You'll find he'll treat you better if you just have more confidence in him."

Here the student has *made a judgment of the patient's feelings and has implied how the patient ought to feel and what he should do.*

Because the student indicated that the patient's feelings were inappropriate, he is unlikely to be free to express other concerns, ask questions about his condition, or be in a position to understand or participate in his treatment.

## The Hostile Response

The patient's comment may well have angered the student. She might then have responded with a comment such as:

"You're certainly not acting very grown up. These doctors know their business. You do an awful lot of complaining about something that you're getting free."

In this instance the student has indicated to the patient not only that his feelings are inappropriate but, in addition, *humiliates* him by implying that he is immature and must accept whatever treatment is given him since the service is free.

## The Reassuring Response

Had the student felt that she should reassure the patient, she might have stated:

"I guess most patients go through a period when they don't understand their doctors. It's really not at all uncommon. I hear that from most patients. But don't worry. He'll tell you eventually."

Here the student has, in effect, *denied that the patient has a problem, and suggests that he need not feel as he does.*

Although denial of his feelings may preclude further discussion (leaving the student with the feeling that the reassurance has *worked*), the patient is no better off than before his talk with the nurse. He remains anxious, confused, worried.

## The Probing Response

Should the student feel that there is some further or hidden meaning in the patient's statement, she might have commented:

"Let's get to the root of your worry. Is there anything else your doctor has done to upset you besides not telling you your diagnosis?"

This type of response implies that if the patient will only *provide more information* the student may be able to provide the answer or solution to his problem. Since a ready-made answer is neither likely nor desirable, the patient is again left prey to his anxiety and misgivings.

## The Understanding Response

An understanding response that would have permitted the patient to express and clarify his feelings might have been: "You're concerned about how sick you really are, and it worries you not to know for sure what your doctor thinks."

Here the student has demonstrated that she is *interested in understanding the patient's point of view, and in communicating that understanding to the patient.*

The patient is more likely to feel safe in such a situation and to sense that whatever attitudes he has are permissible. He may now be free to explore further and modify his feelings toward his physician. Furthermore, the patient, feeling that the student is an understanding person, may be more cooperative in other procedures for which the student may be responsible.

## CONDITIONS FOR EFFECTIVE INTERVIEWING

### Attentiveness

In any interview, the first task is to make the patient as comfortable as possible so that he or she will feel free to express him- or herself. The patient should sense that he or she is the interviewer's sole concern for the duration of the interview.

Attentive and sensitive listening rather than extensive talking on the part of the professional creates a climate in which the patient can communicate. All too frequently we associate the need to help with the need to talk. This association of helpfulness with verbal productivity may well be equated by physicians and nurses with prescribing and "laying on of hands." It must be recognized, however, that it is possible to do something *for* a patient without doing something *to* a patient.

The parodox of "the more listening and the less talking the better" is easily explained. In consulting health workers, a patient is seeking their professional knowledge and skills in relation to physical complaints. Being a recognized expert in this area, the health professional explains and prescribes. During the consultation, the patient may reveal certain related problems. The problems are usually based upon the patient's difficulty, perhaps temporary, in perceiving the situation realistically. Most patients will usually have sufficient inner resources to resolve their difficulties. However, under the stress of illness and perhaps other problems, the patient may experience confusion and conflict. In these cases, the health professional cannot *tell* the patient what to do. The patient must come to understand troublesome feelings independently. Consequently the cardinal rule in interviewing is for the professional to listen more than to talk. This does not imply that the physician or nurse remains passive. The professional's way of listening, which demands skillful participation in the patient's problem solving, is in reality a very active role.

## Attending to Nonverbal Behavior

The interviewer should be aware of and respond appropriately to the patient's complete message, not just to the spoken words. Posture, gestures, blushing, a frown, a smile, a change in tone of voice—these are some of the ways in which people convey relevant feelings. A patient who strikes the table while talking about feelings of anger is dramatically confirming and emphasizing what he has said. On the other hand, nonverbal behavior can deny the verbal message: a patient makes a fist while making a conventional statement of love for family. Since nonverbal behavior is under less conscious control than words, when there is a lack of congruence between the two, the nonverbal message is likely to be more representative of the patient's real attitudes and feelings.

At times, nonverbal behavior is the only communication. For example, a new patient moves about in the chair, looks embarrassed, and appears intensely uncomfortable. The professional who responds to this behavior by saying, "It's very hard for you to get started, isn't it?" will usually ease the situation and elicit an appreciative acknowledgment.

Although some nonverbal behavior may be obvious, interpretation should always be tentative or withheld until the patient verifies it in words or further actions. A frown may indicate annoyance in one person, concentration in another. When the behavior is not clear, there is even more reason to reserve judgment while continuing to note and trying to understand its significance. For example, a woman constantly slips her wedding ring on and off her finger during an interview. The interviewer might hypothesize that the behavior represents ambivalence about her marriage, but will refrain from comment until there is confirming evidence.

Just as the patient communicates nonverbally, so too does the health professional. A patient may frequently look at his watch, implying a wish for the interview to be over; similar behavior on the part of the interviewer is likely to lead the patient to draw the same inference. And the patient, too, is much more likely to believe the nonverbal message when it conflicts with the interviewer's verbal communication.

As interviewers we need to become aware of many minor-seeming aspects of our behavior that affect our patients. For example, various studies have indicated that maintaining eye contact, without "staring down" the patient, conveys a feeling of concern and interest. It may be comfortable for both parties to break eye contact briefly for short periods. Attentiveness is further indicated by a slight leaning forward toward the patient. Leaning back in a reclining swivel chair may communicate that the interviewer's comfort takes precedence over the patient's problems. Posture should be relaxed rather than sitting with arms and/or legs crossed. Patients tend to feel greater anxiety when the interviewer is positioned more than about three feet from the patient. Obviously, extreme proximity can also frighten the patient. There is some evidence that sitting behind a desk may transmit a sense of not being fully available. If the professional sits at the bedside when interviewing a hospitalized patient, rather than standing over the patient, it will contribute to relaxation.

These nonverbal interviewer behaviors have been carefully examined in an investigation at the University of Washington Family Medical Center.[3] The interview portion of 34 initial physician–patient visits was videotaped. Certain nonverbal aspects of the interviewer's behavior (as scored by judges who viewed the tapes) were correlated with patients' satisfaction and patients' understanding of what the physician told them (as determined by postinterview questionnaires). The physician's leaning forward and facing the patient directly made for greater patient satisfaction and understanding. Apparently, the face-on position of the interviewer is perceived by the patient as concern and interest. Touching a patient during the interview was not regarded favorably. Since these were first interviews, touching may have been perceived as somewhat aggressive in an early contact. The sensitive interviewer will become aware of the subtle influences of these easily overlooked matters and, with experience, take increasing responsibility for managing them.

## Note Taking

Record keeping is an integral part of the interviewing process. There are legal and moral responsibilities for maintaining accurate records of all patient contacts. In addition, health professionals will want to review their notes on previous interviews to refresh their memory and to judge progress.

Should notes be taken during an interview or immediately after its termination? Both methods have their supporters. Those who favor note taking during an interview point out that it indicates to the patient that what he or she is reporting is important. Further, for the beginning interviewer, note taking may prevent interruption of a patient's communication. Silences may be more tolerable, since they provide an opportunity to catch up on one's notes.

The present authors favor postponing of note taking until soon after the interview has been terminated. We believe that attentiveness to the patient is lessened if one is also concerned with one's notes. We have observed in the supervisory process that some interviewers interrupt the patient's flow of information and feelings with a request to "Please slow down. I can't keep up with you." Further, it would seem difficult to observe and respond to nonverbal behavior while note taking. Perhaps more important, note taking results inevitably in frequent breaks in eye contact. Interviewers who take only selective notes may inadvertently condition their patients to emphasize those areas that they observe being written down.

Freed of the necessity for note taking, the interviewer can devote entire attention to the patient. Our students report that the intensity of their listening enables them to reconstruct the interview for their later note taking.

The introduction of electronic devices such as audio- and/or videotape in teaching and interviewing situations provides new possibilities and advantages. The tapes can be used to refresh one's memory in reconstructing interviews. More important, listening to and observing one's own interviews provides a constant source of learning and opportunity to improve skills. It is not unusual for interviewers, while listening to their own tapes, to comment on how they might have improved certain responses, or to express the realization that they talked and interrupted too much. As practice continues, the tapes may provide rewarding evidence of the interviewer's improvement.

Ethical considerations require, of course, that the patient's consent be obtained before the recording equipment is used. As in note taking, an explanation should be given before consent is asked. The patient can be told that the purpose of the tapes or notes is to help the interviewer help the patient and that these records can be reviewed to increase understanding of the problem and offer direction for ongoing work together. It should also be emphasized that the material in the notes or tapes will be kept in confidence and used only for purposes of which the patient has been informed and has given consent (eg, teaching, supervision, research). We have yet to experience a refusal of permission under these circumstances. Both patient and interviewer appear to be oblivious to the microphone (the remaining equipment can be kept out of view) several minutes after the interview has begun.

## Preliminaries

Probably each interview will begin with small customary courtesies, such as greetings, the taking of the coat, indicating where the patient may be seated. Most patients will be ready to get to the business at hand. Many physicians and nurses have the mistaken notion that rapport is established by continuing the friendly small talk. To delay "getting on with it" can be burdensome to the patient in pain and can imply that the patient's problems are not taken seriously. Rapport is more likely to be encouraged when the physician or nurse allows the patient to begin discussing matters of concern relatively early in the interview rather than prolonging the small talk.

Rakel[6] recommends, in the interest of furthering rapport, that the health professional review the chart each time before seeing the patient. The purpose of recalling material from the previous visit will ensure follow-up.

## Freedom from Interruption

Attentiveness and rapport can be furthered by freedom from interruption during an interview. Glancing at mail and taking telephone calls will show that you are very busy and much in demand, but they also will demonstrate that you may be too busy to be interested in the patient.

Telephone interruptions in office practice can be handled by asking the receptionist to hold all calls during interviews, except those of dire emergency. If each interview is prefaced by making this request of the receptionist in the presence of the patient, this serves to communicate that the patient is to have the physician's interest for the duration of the interview. A physician who answers his or her own telephone can show the same interest by telling each caller that he or she is presently busy and will call back.

When an interview at the patient's bedside in a hospital is interrupted by a call on the paging system, the physician or nurse can apologize for the interruption and promise the patient to return after answering the page. Of course it is imperative that the professional do so rather than using the page to avoid discussion with the patient.

Should an interview be interrupted by an emergency, it is the health professionals' responsibility to reestablish contact with the patient as soon as possible. They should indicate their regret for the interruption, acknowledge that the patient must have felt "put off," and reschedule the interview for the earliest possible time, preferably when uninterrupted attention can be given.

## Psychologic Privacy

A distinction should be made between *geographic* privacy and *psychologic* privacy for the setting of medical interviews. Perhaps the ultimate in geographic privacy is the comfortably furnished private office sufficiently removed from the waiting room to assure that the interview will be confidential. However, geographic privacy can preclude psychologic privacy if telephone calls or other interruptions are allowed to interfere.

Psychologic privacy does not necessarily demand geographic privacy. In our supervison of medical and nursing students conducting bedside interviews on the large wards of a university hospital, we constantly have been impressed by the psychologic privacy created by merely drawing the curtain between beds. Psychologic privacy can be established in a corner of a hospital lounge, at the end of a corridor, at an obscure table in the cafeteria. The important factors are not geographic. More significant to the patient is the assurance that the interview will not be interrupted or overheard and that the health professional's attitude is one of undivided interest.

## Emotional Objectivity

It is well known that physicians refrain from treating other than minor illnesses in their own families because they are aware that emotional involvement may interfere with the quality of treatment. Objectivity is never easy to achieve. Yet in successful interviewing it is imperative. It goes without saying that objectivity is not equated with coldness. It means, rather, that the interviewer's subjective feelings, likes, and dislikes are under sufficient control that he or she is free to focus on the patient's needs.

It has already been pointed out that the patient must feel free to express not only opinions but also feelings and attitudes. In so doing, the patient may well express notions contrary to those held by the health professional. For example, a patient may reveal to a Catholic physican a decision to obtain a divorce. Or the patient may be critical of persons whom the nurse admires. In some instances the patient may express displeasure with the physician or nurse. Professional workers do not respond as they might in personal situations. They cannot allow themselves the luxury of responding to disagreement or anger in kind. Although this self-discipline may be difficult to achieve, the physician or nurse can be most helpful by continuing to try, even when under attack, to understand why the patient behaves in this way. For example, a hospitalized patient who had grown up in Germany during World War II made repeated antisemitic comments to his Jewish physician. The doctor became inwardly angry each time such statements were made. However, since it would have been awkward to transfer this patient, the doctor attempted to understand why this patient persisted in his remarks. The physician made a tentative inference, which he communicated to the patient. He suggested that the patient was "testing" to see if a Jewish doctor could really accept him. This interpretation served to clear the air and led to the development of mutual trust and respect.

On the other hand is the possibility that the physician and nurse may be unduly influenced by the patient's endorsement of their ideas and attitudes. Or patients may flatter the health professional by their extreme gratitude for what has been done for them. Health workers must be on guard against overtly or subtly encouraging such patients to return to see them, not for medical reasons, but for their own egocentric needs. The mature health professional is motivated by a desire to help patients, not to win their undying gratitude.

## Maintaining the Professional Nature of the Relationship

The health worker must maintain the relationship with the patient at a consistent professional level. Some patients out of gratitude or liking for the professional may wish to develop a more personal contact and extend invitations to their homes, etc. Wise professionals, while refusing such invitations, must be careful not to reject or hurt the patient. They can offer a courteous regret that they cannot accept, explaining that their services must remain professional in the patient's interest, as well as their own. The patient will usually come to see that the professional's judgment is sound and that it will be more comfortable to work with a person who maintains a professional stance.

Expensive gifts can be refused in the same manner and for the same reasons. Acceptance of gifts may create ambiguous and uncomfortable situations. The patient may feel encouraged to make unwarranted demands on the professional, and the professional may feel obligated to accede to these unreasonable requests. Small gifts not intended for any one individual, such as a box of chocolates left at the nursing station, have become acceptable.

## EFFECTS ON PATIENT LOAD, TIME, AND EARNINGS

The question inevitably arises about the demands on health professionals' time if they become concerned with some of the relevant life situations of patients. Will not the time spent reduce the number of patients seen and thus affect earnings?

As to the number of patients seen, McGee[4] points out that each additional patient imposes an added emotional strain on the physician and that errors are likely to be made because of fatigue and the enforced haste of an overloaded practice. He wisely suggests that the physician who functions best is the one who recognizes how many patients the available time and emotional tolerance will allow.

Ferber[2] has interviewed a number of physicians who had introduced a psychotherapeutic concern for patients into their practice. These physicians clearly indicated that patients do not resent a fee for the time taken with them. In some cases earnings increase because less total time is spent with patients. This reduction in time occurs because patients who have had an opportunity for a complete and satisfactory office visit make fewer requests for house calls and other out-of-office demands.

One physician did indicate that his patient load had decreased but added, "I'm seeing fewer patients but giving more time to each one. I still earn all that I want to earn, and I find that it's more satisfying to build my practice around giving all the help I can to every patient I handle" (p. 169).[2]

In general, earnings are not affected. Another physician stated that becoming involved with the personal problems of his patients

". . . hasn't adversely affected my earnings, but even if it did I'd find the satisfaction worth it. There's a point of diminishing returns in how much you can make. But there's no diminution in the satisfaction you get from helping patients and in being able to solve the sort of problems you once thought of as hopeless" (p. 170).[2]

The emphasis was consistently not on reduced earnings but on increased satisfaction. For example, one physician described his work as "the family practice of internal medicine." He perceived his rewards in this manner: "I feel that I'm preventing future maladies as well as dealing with present ones. By trying to understand my patients' family situations as factors in their conditions, I'm dealing with problems that might affect my patients' relatives as well as themselves. In doing so, I'm increasing my patients' comfort and self-awareness, and I'm expanding my own. I'd never go back to any other way of practicing" (p. 170).[2]

## SUMMARY

The interview is the major vehicle for conducting the relationship between health professional and patient. The verbal and nonverbal behavior used by a physician or nurse can be potent forces for therapeutic gain or failure. Social conversational skills must be replaced by a responsible use of communication if the relationship with the patient is to be productive.

Systematic studies of interviewing have shown that virtually every verbal response used in any interaction between people falls into one of five basic categories. In the *evaluative* response the health professional makes a judgment of the patient's feelings and implies what the patient ought to feel and do. The *hostile* response antagonizes or humiliates the patient. It may set in motion a cycle of hostility-counterhostility. In the *reassuring* response one denies, in effect, that the patient has a problem, and suggests that he or she need not feel this way. The *probing* response attempts to elicit more information in order that a ready-made answer to a problem may be provided. The *understanding* response attempts to understand the patient's point of view and to communicate that understanding to the patient. The next five chapters will elaborate on each of these categories of responding.

Basic conditions for effective interviewing were discussed. Attentive listening, including attention to nonverbal behavior, was emphasized as a means for creating a climate in which the patient can communicate. Note taking during the interview may interfere with attentiveness and with responding to the patient's nonverbal behavior, and may lead to frequent interruptions in eye contact. Electronic recording provides excellent opportunity to improve interviewing skills. Rapport is established by demonstrating real interest in the patient and the patient's problems. To continue friendly small talk beyond the courtesy and respect of the usual social amenities may convey to the patient that his or her problems are not taken seriously. As far as possible, interviews should be free from interruptions. Although geographic privacy is desirable for the conduct of an interview, psychologic privacy is essential for providing confidentiality. Emotional objectivity is not equated with coldness and aloofness but emphasizes that the interviewer's subjective feelings are under sufficient control to permit focusing on the patient's needs. It is important for both interviewer and patient that the professional nature of the relationship be maintained. Social invitations, gifts, etc., can be courteously refused with regard to the patient's feelings if realistic and considerate explanation is offered.

The health professional's concern with relevant life situations of patients has no apparent negative effect on patient load or earnings. Fewer requests for house calls and other out-of-office demands are made by the patient who has had a satisfactory office visit. Increased professional satisfaction rather than reduced earnings is the major consequence of a humane practice.

## REFERENCES

1. Bernstein L, Brophy ML, McCarthy MJ, Roepe RL: Teaching nurse–patient relationships: an experimental study. Nurs Res 3:80, 1954
2. Ferber S: The economics of doing psychotherapy. Med Econom 45:106. 1968
3. Larsen KM, Smith CK: Assessment of nonverbal communication in the patient–physician interview. J Fam Pract 12:48, 1981
4. McGee RR: See more patients? There's an emotional limit. Med Econom 48:215, 1971
5. Porter, EH Jr: An Introduction to Therapeutic Counseling. Boston, Houghton Mifflin, 1950
6. Rakel RE: Principles of Family Medicine. Philadelphia, Saunders, 1977

# chapter 3

# The Evaluative Response

## DIAGNOSING AND PRESCRIBING IN ORGANIC ILLNESS AND IN PERSONAL PROBLEMS

The evaluative response has been defined as one in which health workers make a judgment about the patient's feelings, implying what the patient ought to feel and do. In effect, these verbalizations are similar to the medical practices of diagnosing, prescribing, and advising. This process of diagnosing and prescribing is completely appropriate in handling purely organic disease. The man who presents with an infected kidney cannot diagnose his own illness. Neither is he competent to prescribe his own treatment. The physician, with specialized knowledge, is the recognized authority.

Principles underlying the demonstrated effectiveness of physical diagnosis and treatment are stated by Rogers[7] as follows:

1. Every organic condition has a preceding cause.
2. The control of the condition is much more feasible if the cause is known.
3. The discovery and accurate description of the cause is a rational problem of scientific search.
4. The search is best conducted by an individual with a knowledge of scientific method and a knowledge of various organic conditions.
5. The cause, when it is differentiated and discovered, is usually remediable or alterable by materials and/or forces used and manipulated by the diagnostician or his professional associates.

6. To the extent that the alteration of the causative factors must be left in the control of the patient (keeping a diet, restriction of behavior in heart conditions, and so on), a program of education must be undertaken so that the patient perceives the total situation in much the same way as the diagnostician (p. 220).

While these principles have been highly useful in the field of organic illness, not all of them are appropriate for the diagnosis and treatment of psychologic problems. Rogers[7] has indicated that, although psychologic behavior too has a preceding cause, the patient is the only one who can fully know the dynamics of his or her own behavior. Psychologic adjustment is based upon a variety of individual life experiences and not upon anything as specific as a bacterium. Further, identical life experiences do not lead to identical ways of adjusting or coping. For example, one patient about to undergo surgery may openly voice fears and anxieties. Another patient, equally frightened, may put up a brave front so successfully that the fears are not apparent to others.

It follows that there are differences in treating behavioral in contrast to organic problems. As Rogers[7] states this distinction: "The forces which physical medicine can bring to bear, through drugs and other means, appear to have no real counterpart in the psychologic field" (p. 222). Thus penicillin is used to combat a specific organism, but there is no such simple prescription for handling a patient's anxieties. The forces for change in behavior are within the patient, not in some outside agent. It is the health professional's task to help the patient view his or her problems in a new perspective so that these forces for change may be released.

It is apparent that although health professionals can feel quite secure in diagnosing and giving advice in regard to organic illness, these techniques are quite inappropriate in handling a patient's behavioral problems. In using the evaluative response, the health worker may not be far removed from the so-called experts on radio and television or the newspaper columnists who tell people how to solve their problems on the basis of listening briefly or reading a letter.

An evaluative and judgmental attitude may be communicated nonverbally just as effectively as with words. Health professionals are likely to be the recipients of information from their patients relating to crime, sexual deviations, child or wife abuse, and other antisocial behavior. A facial expression of shock or embarrassment can convey disapproval and be just as destructive to the relationship as verbal condemnation.

## The Outcome of Advice Giving

Let us consider the matter of advice giving more concretely. The recipient has two alternatives: to follow the proffered advice or not. Advice is often not followed because the patient senses that the recommended course of action is not appropriate *for him*. Advice is frequently prefaced with "If I were you, . . ." However, the doctor or the nurse is *not* the patient and the recommendation might be quite inappropriate for the individual whose personal dynamics differ markedly from those of the one who is giving the advice. Other patients may fail to follow advice as a means of maintaining their own independence and integrity. These patients feel that by being offered advice they are, in effect, being told that they are incapable of knowing themselves and of working out their own solutions.

Two outcomes are possible if the patient follows the advice: the problem may be solved or it may remain unsolved. If the advice results in solution of the immediate problem, the patient perhaps experiences relief but has learned little or nothing in the process and may also be encouraged in further dependency. The patient may not understand why the advice "worked" and consequently has gained nothing in growth. In fact, growth may have been retarded, and the patient may be no more able to solve new problems as they arise. On the other hand, if the advice is followed but the problem remains or worsens, the patient has been provided with an opportunity to avoid responsibility for his or her behavior, in effect saying "I did as you, the expert, suggested. Therefore, I am not responsible, you are."

## EVALUATIVE AND UNDERSTANDING
## RESPONSES CONTRASTED

In the following incident, advice giving is contrasted with an understanding approach.

As a result of a tragic automobile accident, a second-year medical student was left with a mutilated right hand and arm. The following interchange occurred when, on the day after surgery, the patient revealed his status to the nurse.

PATIENT:
You know, I'm a medical student, a sophomore. I was hoping to be a surgeon. And now this!

NURSE:
I suppose it could have been worse.

PATIENT:
I don't know what I'll do now. . . . I have an uncle in California who is a well-known brain surgeon. (Then bitterly) But how can you be a surgeon with a hand like this?

NURSE:
You may not know it, but you're probably pretty lucky. The real recognition these days comes from medical research, and that's what you should aim for.

PATIENT:
(Angrily) Don't you understand? I said I wanted to be a surgeon! A surgeon, did you hear me?

NURSE:
I was only trying to help.

By offering a gratuitous suggestion, the nurse in this incident seemed to ignore the validity of the patient's grief over his present state of affairs. The advice was probably offered as a means of sidetracking the bitterness being expressed by the patient. Further, she unconsciously may have made the assumption that a second-year medical student did not have either the maturity or the information that would eventually have led him to another specialty. She failed to recognize that the patient would not be ready to think about alternatives until he had worked through his grief.

The nurse was sufficiently upset by this incident to report it to the patient's physician. Contrast the physician's interchange with that of the nurse.

PHYSICIAN:
Good evening, Mr. R. Miss P tells me you're a medical student.

PATIENT:
That bitch!

PHYSICIAN:
Sounds like you two haven't been getting along.

PATIENT:
She's about as warm as an ice cube! I tried to talk to her. Told her about my plans to be a surgeon and she tells me about medical research and recognition. Who wants recognition?

PHYSICIAN:
I guess recognition can't replace your lifelong wish to become a surgeon. Is that what you mean?

PATIENT:
Exactly! I'd want to be a surgeon if it meant being the lowest man on the medical totem pole.

PHYSICIAN:
I can see that you really wanted that.

PATIENT:
I certainly did, and I still do. After my father died, I lived with my uncle in California. He's a neurosurgeon. He treated me like his own son—maybe better. I really admire that man.

PHYSICIAN:
And you wanted to be like him. Even to the point of being a surgeon.

PATIENT:
Right.

At this point the physician was paged and he told the patient he would return. About an hour later the interchange continued.

PHYSICIAN:
Sorry I was so long.

PATIENT:
I'm kind of glad you were. It gave me a chance to think. You mentioned that I wanted to be like my uncle. Well, that's the way it's been. But maybe I should be emphasizing being a good person—generally—like he is. I guess I'd been thinking that if I were a surgeon, I would automatically be like him. But being a surgeon doesn't necessarily mean you're a good guy. It has to be me—as a person, not just a surgeon.

PHYSICIAN:
You want to be like him—surgeon or no surgeon.

PATIENT:
That's it. And to think I blew my stack at that nurse when it was I who was all mixed up! I'll have to apologize to her.

PHYSICIAN:
I'm glad things are looking a little better to you. Well, see you tomorrow.

PATIENT:
Thanks, Doctor.


The physician, rather than giving advice, gave the patient a chance to clarify his feelings. In the process the patient himself gained some insight into his motivation for wishing to be a surgeon. He was not driven into dependency by having the decisions of others foisted on him, and he has had at least one brief experience in trying to solve a new and very difficult problem. This interview illustrates another basic principle of counseling. When an individual faces an overwhelming life situation, as this medical student does, the problems cannot be resolved *in toto,* all at once. They must be broken down and one step considered at a time.

Another point is that the interaction between physician and medical student terminated without any decision as to choice of specialty. Such a choice is not urgent at this time of crisis, and it is probable that the student will arrive at an appropriate decision when he needs to. Even if the interchange had ended at the time the physician was being paged, the outcome would have been similar. The physician's understanding attitude had freed the student to think deeply about his problem.

Frequently health professionals are faced with situations in which an extended relationship may not be possible. Consequently they tend to evaluate the situation quickly and to give advice or direction. This activity may give the health worker the feeling of having helped. However, the patient may be left with poorly understood advice, perhaps resentful, feeling he or she may have done something wrong, and less confident than before. The health professional could instead make use of the limited time to permit the patient to discuss his or her problems and attitudes. As a result the patient may find the problem more clearly defined, with alternatives clarified, and leave with the feeling of being understood and accepted. This feeling, so important to self-esteem, nutures confidence and readiness to tackle problems.

Although it is generally recognized that advice giving is seldom helpful, it is not unusual for patients to make direct requests for advice. The interviewer, who is aware that these requests indicate more of a need to talk of one's problems than a real wish for direction, can handle such requests with comments such as, "You must have given this a good deal of thought. I wonder what *you've* come up with"; or "Could you tell me about the alternatives you've been considering?" The aim of these comments is to encourage the patient to discuss openly his or her own thoughts and feelings about the matter on which advice is sought. As the interviewer helps to clarify these thoughts and feelings, the patient can usually arrive at his or her own decision.

## GIVING INFORMATION

There is an important difference between giving *advice* and giving *information*. In advice giving the health professional usually recommends only one of many alternatives to a patient. The recommended course of action may be based upon insufficient understanding of the patient's problem. For example, the nurse was giving advice when she indicated that the medical student whose hand had been mutilated should seek a career in research as an alternative to surgery. A physician is giving advice in recommending divorce to a patient who complains of a nagging wife.

Information giving, in contrast to advice giving, usually is based upon relatively comprehensive study. Choice is limited to the appropriate action for the specific problem. After taking a thorough history and examining laboratory and x-ray studies, a physician is validly giving information in telling a patient that he or she has an ulcer and should follow a given regimen. A nurse is giving information appropriately in telling a postoperative patient of the need for early ambulation.

One of the most frequent uses of information giving in a medical setting is the prescription of drugs and methods of self-care. It is a serious problem for medical management that there is no assurance that the prescribed regimen will be followed. Many patients do not follow the directions they are given. For example, in a survey of 68 studies of patient compliance, Ley[5] found that nearly 50 percent of patients do not follow the regimens prescribed. Even hospitalized patients often fail to follow medical instructions. It was found that a group of hospitalized patients suffering from peptic ulcer took less than one-half their prescribed antacid. The findings are similar for other types of medical advice, such as dieting and providing vitamin supplements to infants.

These observations led Ley to make a systematic study of the information giving process in a medical setting. He studied 91 patients after their first visit to an outpatient clinic. Between 10 and 80 minutes after seeing the physician, they were asked what they had been told about their illness. Each patient's report was then compared with the physician's record of the diagnosis and instructions to the patient. Surprisingly, one-third of the information could not be remembered. The amount recalled was unrelated to the time elapsed following the medical consultation.

Of the 91 patients interviewed, only 21 (less than 25 percent) remembered everything they had been told by the physician. Furthermore, of these 21 patients who did remember everything, 9 had been given only two items of information. This finding led Ley to reexamine his data to see if there was any relationship between the amount of information given and the amount remembered. Indeed he did find that the more patients were told, the less they remembered. For example, 82 percent remembered everything when given two items of information. When the number of statements received from the physician was three or four, only 36 percent had total recall. If the patient was told five or six things, the percentage of those remembering everything was reduced to 12. If a patient received seven or more statements from the physician, only 3 percent could recall all items.

This finding of an inverse relationship between the amount of information given and the amount remembered has implications for the way in which instructions should be given. It goes without saying that all patients should have clearly written statements of instructions. Further, if the prescribed regimen is to be a complex one, the health professional might begin with one or two items that are likely to give relatively rapid relief. The patient who observes the benefits from this simple compliance will be more likely to accept and follow additional instructions that may make greater demands and take longer to effect results, such as a regular exercise program or modifications in diet. For hospitalized patients, instructions in self-care might start well before discharge and be given in small "doses." Whenever possible, the patient should receive support and encouragement for compliance from the family and from health professionals.

In another study Ley found that twice as many diagnostic statements as instructions for self-care were remembered. Since a physician typically tells the patient the diagnosis first, the observed differential recall may have been related to the tendency of people to remember best what they are told first. To test the latter notion, one group of patients was given self-care instructions before the rest of the information. The result was better recall. Only 43 percent of the instructions were recalled by patients who did not receive them first; those who did receive instructions first recalled 75 percent.

It was found, however, that better recall of instructions led to decreased recall of other material. Consequently attempts were made to find methods of increasing total recall. One such method is based on a finding from experimental work in the psychology of memory: the more easily understood the material, the greater the amount remembered. Using this principle, Ley prepared two versions of a pamphlet intended to motivate obese women to maintain a low-carbohydrate diet. Although both versions had the same content, one was very easy to read (using shorter words and shorter sentences), the other somewhat more difficult. One or the other version was given at random to the subjects in the study. All subjects also received an identical low-carbohydrate diet guide. After a 16-week period, follow-up revealed that those given the very easy pamphlet lost signficantly more weight than those who had the moderately difficult one. Similar results have been found in a different study designed to increase the accuracy with which patients took their medication.

We also know from experimental work that most forgetting takes place immediately after the learning of new material. However, when review occurs soon after the original learning, the amount forgotten is considerably less. The implication for health care is clear. Instruction of patients is not a one-time event. Follow-up shortly after the instruction increases the likelihood of remembering.

Professionals ought not assume, however, that using procedures to improve the patient's memory for self-help regimens will automatically assure understanding and compliance. The professional–patient relationship is particularly relevant in this area. For example, in a study of 800 outpatient visits to the Children's Hospital of Los Angeles,[3] the following results were reported: the mothers' failure to comply with a regimen prescribed for their children was related to the mothers' perception of an unfriendly attitude on the part of the physician and the physician's neglect to explain the diagnosis and cause of the illness. In another study[2] high participation in a pediatric rheumatic fever program was related to the mothers' feeling of being positively evaluated by the clinic staff. Low participation resulted when the mothers felt that the staff disapproved of them. In still another report[1] involving 154 new patients of a general medical clinic in a large teaching hospital, noncompliance was found to be related to unresolved tension in the professional–patient interaction and the failure of the staff to explain why certain information was being asked for.

In some instances a health worker's instructions are ignored, not because they are forgotten or poorly presented, but because they conflict with strong psychologic needs in the patient. This truism will become immediately apparent to the reader who has tried to give up smoking. As long as the consequences of continued smoking remain remote, the need to smoke may persist.

A physician diagnosed emphysema in a 56-year-old man whose chief hobby had been hunting. The physician advised him to give up hunting since the cold air of the north woods aggravated the emphysema. When the patient missed his next appointment because of a hunting trip, the physician wondered what motivation might be so strong as to preclude following instructions crucial for his health. He reasoned that hunting was primarily a man's sport. Since the patient had earlier complained of his waning sexual potency, perhaps giving up hunting constituted a further threat to his masculinity. With this hypothesis in mind, the physician was able, in future interviews, to help the patient accept his aging with less threat, to give up hunting, and to substitute other activities which would satisfy his masculinity needs without threatening his health.

In situations such as these, the health professional should be alert to important psychologic needs that may stand in the way of carrying out self-care instructions. Such needs become readily apparent when a good relationship with the patient has been maintained. The relationship will help the patient and physician discuss and understand how these needs may interfere with good medical management.

Earlier in this chapter, under the heading of "The outcome of advice giving," it was pointed out that people frequently fail to follow advice as a means of maintaining their own independence. One study[4] has demonstrated that if patients can share in decision-making and follow-up responsibility, compliance can be improved. The subjects in this experiment were patients who had been non-compliant after six months of treatment for hypertension. Half of these patients (the experimental group) were instructed in a method of charting their own blood pressure and given a suggested schedule for pill taking at home and fitting their medication into their daily activities. In addition, they were seen every two weeks by a health worker who had no training beyond high school and who offered encouragement and praise for improved compliance and lowered blood pressure. Six months later the control group showed a decrease in compliance of 1.5 percent, while compliance in the experimental group had risen 21.3 percent. Apparently the opportunity to observe the benefits of medication on their self-recorded blood pressures provided the necessary motivation. It can be assumed that the encouragement and praise played their part in the improved compliance.

Of interest in the above study is the fact that it was carried out by a high school graduate, without requiring the time of a busy physician. In another study[8] a nurse interviewed patients in an experimental group following the physician's evaluation. The nurse and patient together filled out a self-treatment form on which were listed the recommendations of the physician, the reasons for the recommendations, and how they should be applied. During the interview the nurse and patient discussed problems that might interfere with following the regimen and how these could be overcome. The control group did not have the interview with the nurse. Two weeks after the initial visit, average patient compliance in the experimental group was 73 percent compared to 55 percent for the control group. Many patients in the experimental group spontaneously commented most favorably about the personal support provided by the nurse, again demonstrating that improved compliance need not take a busy clinician's time.

Finally, it should be pointed out that there is considerable evidence that scare tactics, an overused technique, are usually unsuccessful and may in some cases reduce compliance.[6]

## THE TRAP OF THE QUESTION MARK

Frequently a patient will appear to be asking for advice or information. From experience in ordinary converation, we have learned to respond with an answer to any statement ending with a question mark. Yet not all such questions are really requests for information, and it is important to discriminate those that express an attitude or feeling from genuine information seeking.

In the following interchange, the physician makes this discrimination skillfully:

PATIENT:
I really don't feel any better, doctor. Do you think I should see a specialist?

PHYSICIAN:
You're not satisfied with your progress and are wondering if changing doctors might help.

Physicians are frequently asked questions about their personal lives. Since such questions are not directly related to medical management, the assumption must be made that they most often are expressions of attitude. For example, after relating her problems with her child to a pediatrician, a mother asks:

MOTHER:
Do you have children of your own, doctor?

PEDIATRICIAN:
You doubt whether anyone who is not a parent could really understand your problem.

This understanding statement on the part of the pediatrician creates a climate in which the mother feels she will be understood and therefore can safely continue to discuss her child's problem. The pediatrician who assumed that she was asking for information, and replied with a "Yes" or "No," would have missed this mother's concern.

Student nurses, medical students, interns, and residents are frequently confronted with questions from patients which, in effect, ask whether they are fully trained or are in a learning status. Frequently patients know the answer to such a question before asking it. It appears obvious that patients do not ask these questions "just to make conversation," but to express their doubts about the competence of a person ministering to their needs. A simple, honest statement that they are in fact students merely confirms patients' anxiety. A dishonest denial of their learning status may soon be discovered by patients (if they do not already know it) and lead them to question the accuracy of other information given to them. More appropriate would be an honest answer to the question, followed by a statement showing understanding of the patient's concern. For example, "Yes, I am an intern (student nurse). I can well understand that you have some doubts about how qualified I am to be taking care of you." The patient is then free to ask further questions, which, if also answered in an understanding way, will help ease worry. It will be implicit that the student alone will not carry full responsibility for the patient's care.

In summary, a statement ending in a question mark may be either a request for information or the expression of a feeling or attitude. We have had long training in answering all apparent questions as if they were requests for information. Consequently, in professional situations it will be necessary when questioned to pause and reflect for a moment as to what underlying feeling or attitude may be seeking expression.

## SUMMARY

The evaluative response is one in which health professionals make a judgment of the patient's feelings and imply what the patient ought to feel and do. In effect, they make a diagnosis and prescribe or advise, as in organic illness. However, the principles underlying the effectiveness of diagnosis and prescribing in organic illness do not apply to handling a patient's psychologic problems.

When advice on a personal problem is offered, the patient may follow it or ignore it. Advice may be rejected because of the personal dynamics of the patient. Further, patients may fail to follow advice as a means of maintaining their own independence and integrity.

If advice is followed, the problem may be solved or remain unsolved. In the former case the patient learns little about himself or problem solving and may be pushed into further dependency. If the advice fails to solve the problem, the patient has been provided with an opportunity to avoid responsibility for his or her own behavior.

Even when a patient is given expert information, in contrast to advice, there is no assurance that the prescribed regimen will be followed. Compliance may be improved by beginning with only one or two items of a complex regimen. These first items should be easy to follow and have the likelihood of relatively rapid impact on the patient's condition. More difficult items may then be added. Written and oral directions should be readily understood by the patient. Maintaining a good relationship with the patient is an important determinant in following instructions. One should remain alert to possible psychologic needs that can interfere with compliance. Involving the patient in decision making and follow-up for the prescribed regimen will motivate improved cooperation. Scare tactics have not been effective.

From experience in social conversation, we have learned to respond with an answer to any question. Yet not all such statements are requests for information or advice. The important discrimination to be made is whether a questioner is really asking for information or expressing an attitude or feeling.

## REFERENCES

1. Davis MS: Variations in patients' compliance with doctors' advice: an empirical analysis of patterns of communication. Am J Public Health 58:274, 1968
2. Elling R, Whittemore R, Green M: Patient participation in a pediatric program. J Health Hum Behav 1:183, 1960

3. Francis V, Korsch BM, Morris MJ: Gaps in doctor–patient communication. N Engl J Med 280:535, 1969
4. Haynes RB, Gibson ES, Hackett BC, et al: Improvement of medication compliance in uncontrolled hypertension. Lancet 1:1265, 1976
5. Ley P: Toward better doctor–patient communications. In Bennett AE (ed): Communication Between Doctors and Patients. London, Oxford Univ Press, 1976
6. Matthews D, Hingson R: Improving patient compliance: a guide for physicians. Med Clin North Am 61:879, 1977
7. Rogers CR: Client-Centered Therapy. Boston, Houghton Mifflin, 1951
8. Talkington DR: Maximizing patient compliance by shaping attitudes of self-directed health care. J Fam Pract 6:591, 1978

# chapter 4

# The Hostile Response

## THE HOSTILITY-COUNTERHOSTILITY CYCLE

In Chapter 2 the hostile response was defined as one that antagonizes or humiliates the patient. Such a response may set in motion a cycle of hostility-counterhostility.

Illness frequently leads to regression. Consequently patients are likely to behave in less mature ways than when well. As with young children, they may have a reduced capacity to tolerate delays in having their needs met. They may become irritable and make unreasonable demands on nurses and physicians. In some cases they become openly critical of the professional staff and the care provided. Such behavior tends to make physicians and nurses anxious and resentful. They may retaliate with counterhostility.

Responses to patient hostility were studied in an experimental situation by Gamsky and Farwell.[6] Counselors who were usually understanding persons reacted inappropriately when hostility was directed at them. They became more reassuring and evaluative by giving more information and making more suggestions. It was also found, however, that experienced counselors were better able to withstand hostility than the less experienced.

When health professionals react to patients with counterhostility, a vicious circle may start in which the patient expresses further anger, with the consequence that a professional relationship cannot be maintained. These problems could be avoided if the professional staff recognized that the patient's carping criticisms and angry demands generally are expressions of fear. What the patient is attempting to communicate is worry and confusion about the outcome of the illness and concern over whether the professional staff is doing everything possible to help. This reaction is especially likely when diagnostic procedures are lengthy and initial treatment efforts do not bring immediate changes.

## HOSTILITY AND UNDERSTANDING CONTRASTED

In the following example[1] we see the pitfalls of responding in kind to the hostile statements of a patient:

An elderly patient has returned to the clinic for diagnosis and treatment recommendations. The patient had described her symptoms as similar to those of a previous bout of ulcerative colitis. The physician had done a complete workup the previous week, ordering several laboratory tests and a consultation with a proctologist for a sigmoidoscopy.

PATIENT:
Well, what did you find out about my condition? I certainly hope all those dreadful tests gave you some answers.

The patient's opening comment is a mildly hostile statement, probably related to having been put through the indignities of a sigmoidoscopy.

PHYSICIAN:
Mrs. Fellows, it is not my custom to ask for test procedures or laboratory work that I do not need.

The physician senses the patient's hostility, and begins the hostility-counterhostility cycle.

PATIENT:
Oh, come, Doctor, don't take it personally. You young doctors just grind out orders without thinking what they mean for patients. You knew I had ulcerative colitis, and I knew I had ulcerative colitis, but you still had to ask for all those tests (p. 87).

The physician's overly sensitive and defensive comment brings further criticism from the patient. It might have been more productive to have recognized her feelings about undergoing an unpleasant examination.

After confirming that her ulcerative colitis had again flared, the interview continues:

PATIENT:
I hope I can get over this again. I'd hate to think of living like this

The patient continues her hostile attack by implying that her prethe rest of my life. I had such a good doctor before. Dr. Waggner. You know, he was the most highly respected internist in the city at that time. It's a pity he died so young. But then, I couldn't afford him now, anyway. Well, Dr. Waggner cured me in a matter of months. He just put me on a strict diet and prescribed Pro-Banthine. If you'll write me the same prescriptions, I'm sure I'll be fine.

sent physician is not as competent as her former one. Lacking respect for the clinic physician, she attempts to take over control of her own treatment.

PHYSICIAN:
Mrs. Fellows, if you cannot accept my treatment recommendations you should find a different doctor.

The physician might have responded with, "I can see that you miss Dr. Waggner and that you had a great deal of respect for him." Then he would have avoided competing with her image of her previous physician and her attempt to control the treatment.

PATIENT (begins to cry):
That's easy for you to say! And I wish I could! But I can't afford doctors that really take an interest now. I just have to take whatever you clinic doctors choose to dish out (p. 89).

Although the physician's comment was a statement of his intent to maintain control of the treatment, the hostile manner in which it was communicated was interpreted by the patient as rejection.

In the following example, adapted from Wexler and Adler,[10] the physician successfully avoids the hostility-counterhostility cycle while at the same time laying the foundation for a constructive relationship.

The physician's morning in the ENT clinic has been rather hectic and his appointments are running late. At 10:30 he is ready to see his ten o'clock patient, who has been referred from the Department of Medicine because of difficulties related to equilibrium and hearing. The medical resident's note describes him as a 45-year-old shoe salesman, the father of four, whose symptoms—nausea, vertigo, and tinnitus—sound suspiciously like Meniere's disease. The resident's final comment, "rather irascible—none too pleasant," prepares the physician to expect a difficult, hostile patient.

As the interview begins, the physician's expectations are confirmed. The patient describes his symptoms with an angry, sarcastic edge to his voice. He goes on to state that he has seen three physicians before and received no help from them.

PATIENT:
Those doctors were no damn good.

PHYSICIAN:
(Nods, shows interest, but remains silent.)

By encouraging an angry patient to continue his outburst without limiting the subject matter, he is given an opportunity to express his negative feelings and thereby reduce them. In addition, he is likely to clarify the reasons for his anger.

PATIENT:
Each one gave me a different kind of gobbledygook. One idiot—forgive me—I mean *physician*—suggested that I see a psychiatrist. None of them did me a bit of good. And the way they charged, they must have thought I was J. Paul Getty. I assumed that if you are *forced* to come to a clinic, the charges would be more reasonable.

Had the physician not accepted the patient's hostile feelings (eg, responded instead with, "What do you mean, no damn good?"), the patient may have assumed that the physician was more concerned with a defense of his colleagues than with the patient's interests. Or if the physician had attempted to be reassuring (eg, "This is a new situation and we can start over."), he would have unwittingly asked the patient to sidetrack his feelings. Trying to be encouraging and helpful without recognizing the patient's view usually misfires in the face of so much anger. If he sees his previous experiences with doctors as failures, he isn't likely to accept "Let's let bygones be bygones" with much optimism.

PHYSICIAN:
Forced to come to a clinic?


PATIENT:
Sure, *forced*. I couldn't pay what those other doctors charge even if they could do me any good. I don't have any insurance plan where I work and I can't keep shelling out for doctors or I'll be dead broke. So what can I do but come to a place where I can get cheap help?

By being encouraged to continue on the subject he introduced, the patient has identified one of the factors that may be contributing to his anger, namely, his being "forced" to accept clinic care. Aside from feeling demeaned, he may fear that public care will be inferior to private care.


PHYSICIAN:
You certainly are a very angry man, Mr. Franklin.

By pointing out the patient's anger, the physician indicates that he is willing to deal with these feelings directly.


PATIENT:
You're exactly right, Doctor. I'm mad as hell. Every time I go to a doctor it takes half the day. This morning I cooled my heels a good half hour waiting for you, and I've waited a lot longer for other doctors. At work the manager is complaining that I take too much time off. I try to explain why, but he doesn't give a damn.
Another thing—no one seems to know what's the matter with me. One guy thinks I'm crazy. Another one says I should see a big ear specialist. Maybe I should, but I can't afford it. This noise in my head is going to drive me crazy, if the dizziness doesn't do it first. (The patient appears close to tears.)

It might have been tempting to divert this patient's hostility by beginning to inquire about his symptoms. However, it would have been premature at this point. The emotional climate is still poor and information gathering would be difficult. Further, it would have probably precluded the patient's expression of fear at the end of this statement.

PHYSICIAN:
Perhaps you're more frightened than angry.

The physician recognizes the fearfulness at the conclusion of the patient's last statement and gives the patient an opportunity to discuss and share it.

PATIENT (takes out a handkerchief and blows his nose):
Yes, I guess I am. I don't know what I'm going to do if this gets any worse. It's been going on for about eight months now. Sometimes it gets very bad. . . . Customers sometimes talk to me, and I don't hear what they say. They think I'm being rude. A couple of people complained to the manager. I've got to admit I've gotten more and more irritable—I fly off the handle at most anything. (Long pause.) Listen, I'll try to level with you. I do feel that doctors in clinics are less interested in patients. . . . But I'm willing to start over fresh if you won't hold that against me.

Probably the measure of the physician's success is the patient's frank statement of his feelings about coming to the clinic.
Note, too, that the patient has by now released sufficient anger, and feels sufficiently "safe" so that he himself is suggesting that they "let bygones by bygones."

PHYSICIAN:
I understand. If you feel you are not getting the best care, you can get irritable. . . . Now I need some information, and then I'd like to do a series of ear studies.

By acknowledging and accepting his statement—and neither trying to defend nor to rationalize the type of service provided at clinics—an important step has been taken toward winning this difficult patient's cooperation.

PATIENT:
I'm sorry if I gave you a hard time. (Smiles.) You had every

Whether he changes his mind about doctors and clinics will de-right to throw me out. OK, what do you need to know? (pp. 79–83)

pend as much on how successfully the physician builds on the relationship established with this patient as on the quality of medical care.

## HOSTILITY AROUSED BY "NEUROTIC" PATIENTS

Medical and nursing students receive most of their training in hospitals. Persons with minor illnesses generally are not admitted to hospitals; nor are patients with minimal early signs of what may turn out to be major illness. Consequently nursing and medical students have learning experiences primarily with patients who require specialized diagnostic and treatment procedures. When in practice, physicians and their office nurses are likely to encounter illnesses that they have not met in a hospital. Browne and Freeling[4] have pointed out that, on the basis of hospital training, the physician beginning in general practice may classify patients approximately as follows: 30 percent will be labeled as neurotic, 50 percent as having only trivial illness, 10 percent as malingerers, and only 10 percent as having "genuine" illnesses. The last 10 percent are similar to patients the physician and nurse have seen in their hospital training. Frequently these patients will have to be referred to a variety of specialists. Therefore most of the physician's and nurse's time will be spent with the remaining 90 percent who are not perceived as really ill. Should the physician and the office nurse continue to classify patients in this way, they will probably experience persistent feelings of frustration at the number of patients they regard as neurotic or as presenting trivial complaints. Their frustration will lead to anger, and the anger, however controlled or masked, is likely to be directed, overtly or subtly, at the mass of patients they feel are not worthy of their time and attention.

When no organic basis can be found for their complaints, patients are "reassured" that there is nothing wrong, and frequently are labeled as neurotic, hypochondriac, or the "worried well." These labels represent a rationalization on the part of health professionals for their sense of uncertainty and inadequacy in dealing with such patients. The sense of rejection aroused in patients who have received this pseudodiagnosis, which does not, after all, change or end their complaints, may lead to a frustrating round of "doctor shopping" or, as previously indicated, detour to quacks.

Physical symptoms represent a socially approved method of seeking and receiving "care" from one's family, friends, and health professionals. Hence, it may be said that somatization has been learned as a method for expressing psychosocial stress. Rosen et al[9] suggest the need for a change from the biomedical model of illness, in which the diagnostic process is completed when an organic basis has been ruled in or out, to a biopsychosocial model, in which social and cultural aspects of illness are considered legitimate health-care problems.

Barton[2] suggests that the neurotic or hypochondriac label is used when the health professional perceives certain suggestive personality characteristics in the patient. He goes on to point out that, if understood, these signs could become valuable diagnostic suggestions, indicating the need for exploration of the broader psychologic aspects of illness. If symptoms are viewed as a form of interpersonal communication, it may turn out that the patient who reports pain and pressure in the epigastrum is really complaining of a painful experience on the job or in the family. For example, a physician could find no organic basis for a patient's complaint of excruciating abdominal pain. The patient appeared disappointed when hospitalization was not recommended. Rather than dismiss this patient, the physician encouraged discussion of the events preceding his attack. Soon he was able to disclose that the sudden onset of pain had interrupted his wife's preparation to leave him. Instead, she brought him to their physician's office. The patient was able to see the possible connection between his symptoms and his need to prevent his wife from leaving him. Subsequently a referral to marriage counseling was accepted by both partners. To label this patient neurotic would ignore the fact that he suffers from his symptom just as surely as a patient with a "genuine" illness. To dismiss patients as neurotic because their symptoms have no organic basis is akin to refusing to treat patients with terminal illness because they cannot be cured.

## HOSTILITY EXPRESSED AS HUMOR

Hospital "shop talk" has many catch phrases that offer the relief of humor to the "in" group but often seem callous to others. The chronic neurology ward is referred to as "the vegetable garden." The autopsy conference becomes "man-in-the-pan rounds." The obsessive-compulsive patient is characterized as "excessive-repulsive." Advice for treating the dying patient is "Give him a Bible and tell him to cram for the final."

The development of such expressions is understandable. The physical environment of the hospital has been described as one of deformity, pus, and excreta; the emotional environment, as one of pain, unhappiness, and anxiety.[4] Persons in the health professions tend to develop certain protective mechanisms in an attempt to make this grim reality more tolerable. Frequently these mechanisms take the form of hostile humor. Wit involves a clever play on words or meanings to give temporary relief from the strain of reality.

When patients or their relatives overhear such remarks, the damage to the professional relationship is inevitably severe. Deaton[5] has made this observation:

> The medical profession loses face every time a hospital physician is overheard making a careless remark. When doctors drop their guard, patients and their relatives have an uncanny way of being in the corridor, or near the nurse's station, or next in line in the cafeteria. It's almost axiomatic, too, that when something indiscreet is said about a patient within hearing distance of a stranger, that stranger will turn out to be the patient's closest relative. While in the hospital, patients—and their visiting relatives—have the state of the patient's health foremost in their minds. Since they know that the doctor is the best source of information on that subject, it's no wonder that he draws them like a magnet. So, if he uses such expressions as "that poor slob" or "that old crock in 714," the chances are all too good that the wrong person will be nearby. To keep from saying something that the next minute he'd pass up a two-week conference in Hawaii to unsay, the hospital physician has to be on his guard all the time. It's the only preventive I know for foot-in-mouth disease (p. 58).

These comments apply equally to nurses. The following incident was reported to us:

NURSE A:
I heard Mr. B was admitted again

NURSE B:
Oh, yes, the old kook came in last night.

NURSE A:
Anything the matter with him, or did he have a fight with his wife again?

NURSE B:
Oh, she's probably tired of having him around and sent him in for the winter.

NURSE A:
Why don't you get hold of Dr. S and see if you can't get the old buzzard out?

NURSE B:
That's a good idea. No need of him being here taking up a bed.

Next day the patient (Mr. B) asked to be discharged against medical advice, stating that he had urgent business elsewhere. An aide was told by another patient that Mr. B left because he had overheard the above conversation.

## HOSTILITY USED TO DENY DEPRESSION

McMahon and Shore[8] have described the emotional responses of fourth-year medical students at Tufts University School of Medicine, while they were making house calls in deteriorated sections of the inner city of Boston. Most students were depressed by these experiences. (Nursing students making public-health or visiting-nurse visits in the slums would probably show similar reactions.) One method used to deny their depression was to become rejecting and punitive toward these patients. The students characterized these disadvantaged patients as ". . . irresponsible, self-indulgent schemers who were cheating the taxpayers by manipulating welfare" (p. 564).[8] They recommended cutting off aid to illegitimate children, forcing the recipients of welfare to work, and separating children from their parents.

Interestingly, these attitudes toward the poor appear to be related to certain similarities between the circumstances of students and their indigent patients. Students preparing for the medical professions are likely to be supported by parents or spouses, resulting in an economic dependency that may threaten their sense of adequacy and maturity. "It was not difficult to see what lay behind these students' envious phantasies that the poor were leading libertine lives, making money off AFDC [Aid to Families with Dependent Children], by sexual indulgence, surrounded by color television and Princess phones, free of responsibility" (p. 564).[8]

The punitive, rejecting attitudes of the students interfered with successful functioning in these situations. Their perceptions were so distorted that they failed to see social and economic factors that were perhaps beyond the patients' control. Their rejection precluded the development of an understanding professional relationship. Anger led to retaliation against those who did not follow instructions, who missed appointments, or who presented trivial complaints. The retaliation manifested itself in inappropriate and aggressive methods of treatment. For example, one student administered intramuscular injections for a febrile illness for which oral penicillin was indicated. He rationalized that the patient was too ignorant and uncooperative to follow an oral dosage regimen.

## TRANSFERENCE AND COUNTERTRANSFERENCE

### Transference

As the nurse–patient or physician–patient relationship develops, patients tend to regard these health professionals as authority figures and to invest them with the characteristics of good or bad parents. This phenomenon is known as *transference*. Transference is the process whereby feelings of love, hatred, trust, and distrust that were originally attached to significant persons in the past (usually parents) are displaced or projected unconsciously onto important individuals in the present. In other words, transference indicates how the patient perceives health professionals and influences the patient's behavior toward them. If the relationship is a good one, we refer to a positive transference; if the patient's feelings are those of hostility and fear, the transference is negative.

We shall be concerned in this chapter primarily with negative transference. Typically, positive transference presents fewer problems since it is usually synonymous with a positive professional–patient relationship. In fact, the transfer elements are usually not apparent or intrusive in a good relationship between mature adults. When the positive feelings become inappropriate (for example, when a patient wishes to have a social relationship with the nurse or physician), however, these feelings will have to be discussed frankly and openly. It can be explained to the patient that such feelings frequently develop in an understanding and helping relationship. Usually these feelings diminish with time. In any case, the health professional's responsibility is to clarify differences between personal and professional relationships without rejecting the patient.

Negative transference is encountered when a patient tests the professional worker's sincerity by repeated criticism, unrealistic expectations, or aggressiveness. In a medical setting it is, in fact, difficult to escape becoming the target of a barrage of negative, hostile, angry emotions. Professionals need to understand that such feelings are rarely of their making. They are perhaps patients' generalized mode of reacting to those in authority or to those associated with the uncomfortable circumstances of the illness. From their experience in usual family and social relationships, patients expect hostility to be met with counterhostility. If health professionals choose not to respond defensively or angrily and do not use authority to browbeat, belittle, or maintain distance from patients, they avoid the risk of perpetuating the hostility-counterhostility cycle. When health workers realize that although negative feelings are displaced onto them, they are not necessarily aroused by them, they will be free to react understandingly rather than aggressively. Then patients are likely to modify their negative behavior. Eventually patients are able to perceive that under certain circumstances they need not fear counterhostility when their anxiety and anger exceed their control. Under these conditions the patient's relationship to the nurse or physician can develop in the positive direction necessary for optimal progress.

## Countertransference

Just as the patient projects feelings from past relationships onto the nurse or physician, the nurse and physician experience similar reactions to patients. This process is labeled *countertransference*. Every individual, no matter what his or her status, has prejudices, immaturities, objects of disgust, and punitive tendencies derived from life experiences. If members of the health team lack self-awareness, their responses to patients may be influenced by their own feelings to the detriment of the professional–patient relationship and may jeopardize the outcome of treatment.

An illustration of such countertransference is provided by Browne and Freeling.[4] They report a physician's difficulty in dealing with parents of adolescent patients he was treating for acne. Upon reflection, this doctor became aware that he was able to give friendly attention to adolescents with acne when they came to his office by themselves, but he became highly irritable when they were accompanied by their mothers. He recalled his own adolescent acne for which he had been taken by his own mother from one physician to another. Although his skin condition was of no concern to him, his mother required him to give up many of his favorite foods and to follow cleansing and rest routines, which he disliked. When he became aware that he was reacting to his young patients on the basis of his own adolescent experience, this physician was able to improve his handling of such cases.

Similarly a psychiatric nurse found herself constantly questioning diagnoses of schizophrenia in patients with a history of alcoholism. She had no problem, however, in accepting a diagnosis of schizophrenia in patients in whom alcoholism was not a factor. When this distinction was pointed out to her, she was able to reveal a very close relationship with her own father, who had been an alcoholic for many years. More recently her father had been committed to a state hospital as a schizophrenic, a fact which caused her much anguish and guilt.

Countertransference phenomena occur frequently enough to suggest that professional health workers need to examine, as honestly and objectively as possible, their emotional reactions to patients. Most health professionals, upon reflection, will discover that certain kinds of patients arouse negative feelings. Some find it difficult to work with alcoholics, some with the aged or with the overly dependent patient, and so on. They find themselves treating such patients with less respect and patience. That professional people respond in this profoundly human way is not surprising. It is detrimental, however, if self-examination is avoided or spontaneous reactions denied. Self-scrutiny may be of help to many health professionals in overcoming these spontaneous reactions. In some cases, however, it may be necessary to avoid working with those who consistently arouse negative feelings. For others, the solution for countertransference problems that interfere with the physician–patient or nurse–patient relationship may be personal psychotherapy.

When one becomes aware that countertransference feelings may have interfered with communication with patients, the physician or nurse should attempt to identify the source of such feelings. The following list of questions, adapted in part from Brammer and Shostrom[3] and from Lawton,[7] may be useful in understanding why communication has broken down:

1. Do I require sympathy, protection, and warmth so much myself that I err by being too sympathetic, too protective toward the patient?
2. Do I fear closeness so much that I err by being indifferent, rejecting, cold?
3. Do I need to feel important and therefore keep patients dependent on me, precluding their independence and assuming responsibility for their own welfare?
4. Do I cover feelings of inferiority with a front of superiority, thereby rejecting patients' needs for acceptance?
5. Is my need to be liked so great that I become angry when a patient is rude, unappreciative, or uncooperative?

6. Do I react to the patient as an individual human being or do I label him or her with the stereotype of a group? Are my prejudices justified?
7. Am I competing with other authority figures in the patient's life when I offer advice contrary to that of another health professional?
8. Does the patient remind me too much of my own problems when I find myself being overly ready with pseudo-optimism and facile reassurance?
9. Do I give uncalled-for advice as a means of appearing all-wise?
10. Do I talk more than listen to a patient in an effort to impress him or her with my knowledge?

Although this checklist will not preclude all countertransference phenomena, thoughtful review of these questions will increase self-awareness. A heightened consciousness of their own behavior will help health professionals to avoid potentially harmful reactions to patients.

## SUMMARY

The hostile response antagonizes or humiliates the patient. Such a response may start a cycle of hostility-counterhostility, which could be avoided if health professionals recognized that generally the patient's criticisms and angry demands are expressions of fear or anxiety.

Since medical and nursing students receive most of their training in hospitals where they see, for the most part, serious disease, they regard many of the illnesses seen in later practice as trivial or neurotic. Their frustration can lead to anger toward these patients. Trivial complaints should not be taken lightly. They may be diagnostic leads to other illness and, in addition, may provide an entree to symptom-causing concerns that the patient has difficulty discussing.

The expression of hospital "shop talk" in the form of hostile humor offers health professionals some relief from the realities of pain and suffering. To patients and their relatives, however, this hostile wit appears callous. Members of the health team must be constantly on guard against having such humor overheard.

Rejecting and punitive attitudes are used frequently as a means of denying the depression health professionals experience when working with disadvantaged or desperately ill patients.

*Transference* is the process whereby a patient's feelings, which originally were attached to significant persons in the past, are displaced or projected onto the nurse or physician. If the relationship between health professional and patient is a good one, we refer to *positive* transference; if the patient's feelings are anger and fear, the transference is *negative*.

Typically, positive transference presents no major problems. When the patient's positive feelings become overly intense, however, they will have to be discussed openly and frankly without rejecting the patient. A patient who demonstrates negative transference, expects hostility to be met with counterhostility. If the physician or nurse reacts with understanding, the patient's expectation is not reinforced and the negative behavior is likely to be modified.

Just as the patient projects feelings from past relationships onto the physician or nurse, the physician and nurse experience similar reactions to patients. This process is labeled *countertransference*. Health workers need to examine as honestly and objectively as possible their emotional reactions to patients to avoid potentially destructive professional behavior. Such self-scrutiny may help overcome countertransference reactions. In some cases it may be necessary to avoid working with categories of patients who consistently arouse negative feelings. For some, countertransference feelings may be clarified in personal psychotherapy.

# REFERENCES

1. Adler LM, Wexler M: Winning the patient's confidence in your treatment. Hosp Physician 5:86, 1969
2. Barton D: Patient labels in medical practice. N Physician 21:360, 1972
3. Brammer LM, Shostrom EL: Therapeutic Counseling, 2nd ed. Englewood Cliffs, Prentice-Hall, 1968
4. Browne K, Freeling P: The Doctor–Patient Relationship. Edinburgh and London, Livingstone, 1967
5. Deaton JG: "That crock in 714" may be listening. Hosp Physician 3:56, 1967
6. Gamsky NR, Farwell GF: Counselor verbal behavior as a function of client hostility. J Counsel Psychol 13:184, 1966
7. Lawton G: Neurotic interaction between counselor and counselee. J Counsel Psychol 5:28, 1958
8. McMahon AW, Shore MF: Some psychological reactions to working with the poor. Arch Gen Psychiatry 18:562, 1968
9. Rosen G, Kleinman A, Katon W: Somatization in family practice: a bio-psychosocial approach. J Fam Pract 14:493, 1982
10. Wexler M, Adler LM: Winning the hostile patient's cooperation. Hosp Physician 5:78, 1969

# chapter 5

# The Reassuring Response

In Chapter 2 we discussed the differences between social conversation and professional interviews. In a social interchange, one of the most common ways of handling the expression of negative feeling or anxiety is through reassurance, usually pat or cheerful phrases in the face of disturbing events. When a patient expresses a fear of impending surgery, for example, it is not uncommon to hear the bromides: "Cheer up, don't worry about it," or "Everything is going to be all right." As far as the patient is concerned, such reassurance is not only gratuitous but possibly harmful.

## THE NEGATIVE ASPECTS OF REASSURANCE

### Reassurance Denies That a Problem Exists

When a patient has given vent to fears, being "soothed" with "things will work out all right" or "everyone feels that way just before surgery" amounts to a statement that the problem does not exist or it is not serious. Such responses deny the patient's feelings and make it difficult to explore concerns more fully. A patient is not likely to reveal anxieties when it has been implied that they do not or should not exist. Reassurance cannot change the fact that they do exist.

A medical resident submitted the following incident to the authors for evaluation:

Patient came to my office this morning apparently wanting to talk.

PATIENT:

I know you folks have done all you can for me, and I want you to know I appreciate it, but I don't think I will get any better. (Patient had tears in his eyes and was quite depressed.)

Patient is expressing his discouragement over his rate of progress.

RESIDENT:

I am sure you will soon feel better. (I tried to ward off any further conversation.)

What evidence does the resident have that the patient "will soon feel better"? This statement is indicative of his wish to discourage discussion of the patient's feelings, as indicated in the parenthetical comment.

PATIENT:

No. I'm not getting along with my wife, and I feel that it is all my fault, since I have broken down before. I don't want to hurt her any more.

In spite of the resident's denial of the problem, the patient tries again to communicate his worry. He reveals a marital problem related to his own feelings of discouragement.

RESIDENT:

Uh—I don't think your wife feels that way. I am sure that you will be able to straighten things out after you feel better.

Again the resident resorts to denial. How can he know how the patient's wife feels?

PATIENT:

Well, I don't know. (Mr. G walked away very dejectedly.)

After two attempts, the patient gives up. The fact that he "walked away very dejectedly" indicates that denial of the patient's feelings did not change them.

To this resident's credit was his recognition that this was not a helpful interchange. He noted that the patient "walked away very dejectedly," and he therefore submitted this incident for review. He might have let himself believe that his reassurance "worked" since the patient left the office so quickly.

## Reassurance Does Not Really Reassure

The superficiality of the reassurance in the above incident is immediately apparent, as is the resident's discomfort with the patient's depression. Even when the physician or nurse sincerely feels confident and optimistic, however, the patient cannot be made to share these feelings by a "pep talk." Rather, the patient can achieve assurance from an opportunity to explore and understand his or her feelings. As Gregg[2] has stated,

> . . . patients feel reassured when they are helped to use their own skills to work with problems that seem overwhelming at the outset. Patients probably feel reassured when someone is willing to listen and to value them as persons, accepting what they say without condemning them for expressing what they feel (p. 173).

The following incident, reported to us by a nurse, is illustrative:

Mr. X was a new patient who had been admitted to the medical service with a probable bleeding ulcer.

PATIENT:
I guess this might be the end for me. I'm 57 now. I guess I could go any time.

NURSE:
You're afraid that if you're sick enough to come to the hospital, you might die.

Although the mention of fear of dying frequently elicits reassurance, the nurse chose to reflect the patient's concern, rather than reassure him.

PATIENT:
Well, lots of people die when they get this old. I guess I might have cancer, don't I?

Sensing that the nurse was accepting his feelings, even the fear of death, the patient felt safe in revealing that his concern was with cancer.

NURSE:
You are worried that your bleeding may have been caused by cancer.

The nurse skillfully avoided the "trap of the question mark." Instead, she continued to communicate her understanding of the patient's concern.

PATIENT:

Well, I don't see what else it could be. (Short pause.) Of course, I have been pretty healthy all my life. And I don't have the other symptoms that go along with cancer. I eat well and I haven't lost any weight.

After the opportunity to express his fear, the patient was able to modify his feeling, recognizing that his fears were exaggerated. Additional discussion, exploring further the realities of his health condition, might have been beneficial.

## Reassurance Protects the Health Professional's, Not the Patient's, Feelings

Health care personnel often say that they use reassurance to prevent the patient's anxiety from getting out of control. One might surmise that this explanation is frequently a rationalization. The patient, by exposing feelings, has indicated a desire to discuss them. A reassuring response suggests that health workers would prefer not to discuss such matters, perhaps leaving the patient with the distressing feeling of having raised inappropriate concerns. On the contrary, however, the professionals may well be avoiding material difficult for them. Health care personnel should ask themselves, when tempted to reassure a patient, whether they are protecting themselves or the patient. If they are honest, they will in most cases recognize that they are attempting to avoid discussion of a matter that would make them uncomfortable.

## FALSE REASSURANCE

We can conclude then that attempts to reassure by such statements as, "There is no reason to worry," or, "Cheer up, everything will be all right," are quite ineffective. They do not work because they rely on spurious methods to ease or quiet the patient—falsification, changing the subject, or avoidance.

## Falsification

A pediatrician approaches a hospitalized child to administer an injection. To gain the child's cooperation the pediatrician says, "This won't hurt." Trustingly the child submits. The pediatrician believes the reassurance has been successful since the injection was given without major incident. What was ignored at the time was that an additional injection would be required the following day. The child, seeing this doctor approach again, runs down the corridor and hides in the linen closet. The pediatrician writes in the progress notes: "Child is uncooperative today." It might have been more accurate if the entry had read: "I lied to this child yesterday, and the child is on to me today."

Falsification frequently is used to explain the absence of a patient who has died. To avoid discussion of death, other patients are told by the nurse or other ward personnel that the dead patient was transferred to another ward. It is well known that patients soon discover the truth. One wonders to what extent a patient will trust other information given by a nurse (or physician) who has resorted to such falsification. A lie merely postpones discovery of the truth. When the truth is discovered, the situation will be more difficult to handle. This awkward circumstance would not have arisen if the health worker had recognized the anxiety behind the question in the first place and responded accordingly.

A flagrant use of falsification occurred during a bedside interview by a medical student. The patient broke into tears after telling him she could no longer have children following recent surgery. Her surgeon had told her he would remove one tube but found it necessary to tie the other as well. The student's extreme discomfort in the face of this woman's open distress led him to say, "I'm sure he wouldn't have done it if he didn't believe it necessary. And, if I remember correctly, we were told in class yesterday that it is now possible to have children even after the tubes have been tied. Why don't you talk to your doctor about it when he comes around?" This statement served the student's needs very well. The patient stopped crying and the student left the room. The student did avoid a "scene." What of the "scene" the following day, however, when the patient's surgeon confronted the student with the "facts of life"? This incident may have had even further implications. Might the patient be confused by contradictory information from two different "authorities"? Or could she have felt that possibly the medical student had more recent information than her busy practicing surgeon? If so, how would the physician–patient relationship have been affected?

## Changing the Subject

A technique used primarily to protect the health worker's feelings rather than the patient's is changing the subject to something more pleasant. For example, a nurse reports: "A patient with a poor prognosis asked me if I thought he would ever get well. Not knowing how I could discuss his progress honestly, I told him it was about time for his dinner tray to come, and he might enjoy his meal more if I first straightened his pillows and rubbed his back. While doing so, I interested the patient in talking about travel in Colorado." To allay her discomfort the nurse resorted to physical care and changed the subject to something about which *she* felt more comfortable. The patient's concern was ignored.

Similarly when a patient says that he or she feels like dying and the physician responds with, "Did you enjoy your visitors over the weekend?" a desire is indicated to close a subject that is too disturbing. Wolberg[3] points out that introducing irrelevant material to distract the patient from painful areas interferes with modification of feelings; dealing with feelings and attitudes facilitates modification. Consequently health professionals must sensitize themselves to immediate feelings and not divert the patient by introducing irrelevant topics or asking unrelated questions.

## Avoidance

The professional persons' most extreme tactic for protecting themselves from unpleasant situations or discussions is to stay away from the patient as much as possible. Although the terminally ill patient is the one most likely to be avoided, health professionals also tend to stay away from patients who are upset, demanding, and hostile. When avoidance is practiced, the patient experiences isolation and loneliness but is not reassured.

In discussing the handling of the dying patient by hospital staff, Glaser and Strauss[1] point out that:

> Physicians and nurses understandably develop both standardized and idiosyncratic modes of coping with the worst hazards. The most standard mode—recognized by physicians and nurses themselves—is a tendency to avoid contact with those patients who, as yet unaware of impending death, are inclined to question staff members, with those who have not "accepted" their approaching deaths, and with those whose terminality is accompanied by great pain (p. 5).

Not only are patients avoided, but relatives are insulated in "distant waiting rooms, offices, or main lobbies to wait out the crisis" (p. 232).[1] Although relatives are frequently told that they will be in-

formed of changes in the patient's condition, the physician or nurse
may conveniently forget to do so. "Forgetting, like avoiding, is a standard strategy for maintaining composure" (p. 233).[1]

Complete avoidance of emotional involvement with the patient is
possible only when the patient is comatose or heavily sedated. With a
patient who is alert "expressive avoidance" is used:

> . . . they avoid him as a person while they are fulfilling their
> medical duties. They ignore him, treat him as a body (that is,
> socially dead), wear bland professional facial expressions, ex-
> ude dignity and efficiency, and refuse or evade conversation,
> or else do their chores quickly and "get out" before the patient
> can say anything (p. 237).[1]

The major consequence of such strategies is that the patient loses
trust in the physician and/or nurse; ". . . and this in turn may make
[them] less effective in patient care and unnecessarily hard on the
patient and his family" (p. 251).[1]

## REASSURANCE AND UNDERSTANDING CONTRASTED

The following incident, adapted from Gregg,[2] points up the differences
in patient care resulting from the use of false reassurance as contrasted with an understanding approach.

A resident walked into a patient's room and found her looking
very forlorn and upset. Their conversation was as follows:

RESIDENT:
Oh, come now, Mrs. Carson, nothing could be that bad! You look
like you've lost your last friend!

Mrs. Carson's unspoken reaction
to the resident's comment might
have been: "I feel very upset, and
he can see that I am upset. Why
does he say, 'Nothing could be
that bad'? How could he possibly
know?"

Such clichés frequently are used
to reduce the danger of an un-
wanted "scene" and to preserve
social equanimity. They also re-

duce the importance of the other person's feelings.

PATIENT:
My doctor just told me that it will be impossible for me to get well if I don't have the operation. I'm so mixed up—I wish I knew what to do.

RESIDENT:
There is only one thing to do and that is to have the surgery! You haven't a thing to worry about. You have the best surgeon in town. He has done hundreds of operations just like yours.

The patient's feelings about the resident's second comment might have been: "I tried to tell him I was mixed up. It is hard for me to explain how I feel, and he didn't even let me finish! He thinks I am frightened about the operation. I guess he wouldn't know what it's like to be afraid of something bigger than an operation! What does he mean—'I haven't anything to worry about'? I wonder what he would do if he had my little boy? He doesn't even know what I'm worried about! Maybe that's it— maybe he doesn't want to know. I guess I really shouldn't bother other people with this. No one could possibly understand how I feel."

This woman's probable, if unexpressed, reaction of anger and confusion is one possible outcome of jumping ahead of a patient's communication and guessing at what she is trying to say. The guess can easily be wrong and, furthermore, it conveys that what the patient has to say is not important.

The resident's emphatic recommendation that the patient

should go ahead with surgery seems, at best, gratuitous. The decision is not his to make. He cannot know what doubts or other problems the patient must first resolve, since she has not yet had an opportunity to reveal them.

PATIENT:

You don't understand—I have confidence in my doctor—it's—well—

RESIDENT:

Most people are a little scared when they think about having an operation. Remember when you had your first baby several years ago when I was a medical student working on OB? You had the longest and hardest labor of anyone on the ward, and I never heard a whimper out of you! I was so proud of you! You were the best patient in the whole hospital! After what you went through, this operation should be a picnic, and this time you'll be completely unconscious from the anesthetic. You won't feel a thing.

This "speech" may have made the patient feel: "He didn't let me finish—he must think I am stupid because I can't talk without stumbling over my words. There he goes again about the operation. What is this about the birth of my baby? If he only knew—I was so scared I couldn't whimper—but *he* was proud of me! That baby is my biggest problem! Oh, what's the use? How could anyone understand about John? He says I won't feel a thing—maybe I won't—maybe I really won't. Anyway, I'm supposed to keep quiet."

As she hesitated and searched for words, the resident became anxious and again guessed at her problem, thereby cutting off the patient's attempt to talk about what was really bothering her. Further, he unwittingly told the patient how he expected her to behave by praising her past performance. He also attempted a perhaps irrelevant reassurance by saying the coming episode would be a "picnic." It is rarely comforting to an anxiety-ridden person to be told that she will be unconscious, for, in her apprehension, she may find this state simply another situation in which she will be "out of control."

Later in the day, the nurse entered the same patient's room during evening rounds. Mrs. Carson smiled a greeting but initiated no conversation. She seemed preoccupied, and her face was tear-stained.

NURSE:
It seems hard for you to relax tonight. You must have had a difficult day.

In this statement, the nurse recognized the patient's distress, as did the resident in the first episode. In contrast, however, she did not make light of the patient's feelings. She offered an opening for the patient to communicate her distress, which the discouraged patient seemed disinclined to take.

PATIENT:
Yes. (Silence.)

NURSE:
Feel like talking about it?

With this statement, the nurse provided further opportunity for the patient to speak. To be helpful, this question would have to reflect the nurse's sincere interest. If it were mere curiosity, the patient would probably have sensed it as such. The nurse observed that the patient was disturbed but, at this point, needed help to talk and to feel that the nurse would actually listen to her.

PATIENT:
It would seem silly to you. It's so hard to explain. If I thought I could make it home, I would leave—. No one understands.

The patient here gave three clues to the fact that it would be difficult for her to feel accepted enough to talk about her problem: (1) she expected the nurse to think that her distress was silly; (2) she said that her feelings were hard to explain; and (3) she wished to escape the whole issue by going home.

NURSE:
I'll try to understand, if it will help.

This simple but highly emphatic statement accomplished several purposes. The nurse conveyed to the patient that she wanted to understand, even though the patient thought that was impossible. She also seemed to understand that the patient's idea of avoiding surgery and going home was more in the nature of a desperate "escape" from her difficulties than a final decision.

PATIENT:
They say I have to have an operation, and I'm so scared and mixed up. They think it's the operation that scares me, but—oh, well—I don't know how you could understand. I'm in such a mess! (Silence.)

NURSE:
It's hard to explain.

This statement was an attempt by the nurse to identify and accept the patient's feeling of half-wanting and half-not-wanting to talk it over, and to show that she accepted the turmoil that the patient felt.

PATIENT:
Yes—if I weren't around maybe he could get someone who would really help John. I just don't have the patience any more. Maybe I never did! (Pause.)

NURSE:
Could you tell me who John is, and who could get someone else?

The nurse's request for clarification achieved two purposes: (1) she conveyed that she was really interested in knowing exactly what was being said, and (2) she helped the patient communicate more clearly. Issues are often perceived more clearly as they are explained to another person.

PATIENT:
John is my son. He has cerebral palsy. He is a sweet little boy but he needs so much care, and you have to be so patient, and I'm just not. Since I've been sick, we haven't been able to send him to his special school. My medical bills stand in the way of his chance to get help, and when he is home all the time—well—I guess I get impatient with his troubles, and I'm always scolding when I know he can't help it. My husband has the burden of both of us. He is so kind to the boy, and so patient with me. They would both be better off without me. I shouldn't have the operation.

NURSE:
Are you saying that you may not live if you don't have the operation and that it would be better for John and your husband?

In seeking further clarification, the nurse used a slightly different method. She focused on something the patient said and tried to help her reexamine it to see if she really meant what she was saying.

PATIENT:
The doctor said I can't expect to live long without surgery. (Thoughtful silence.) I guess I really am silly—that would be kind of like suicide, wouldn't it? (Crying.) Now you know how mixed up I am! I guess I am a little crazy—worrying about John and the money and everything. (Sobbing.)

Within an accepting relationship, the patient was able to take the next step in problem solving. Mrs. Carson took a second look at what her death would mean. As she realized somewhat more clearly what she had been thinking, she became self-condemnatory, crying and saying she was "mixed up" and "crazy."

NURSE:
(hands patient a facial tissue): It's such a tough problem that you would like to escape from it.

The nurse's behavior indicated that it was all right for her to feel and act upset. She sympathetically realized with her that hers was indeed a difficult situation. This acceptance made it possible for the patient to explore her feelings further and uncover more facets of the problem.

PATIENT:
Yes, but I don't really want to die. I can't really say that my husband would be better off if I died. He would be all alone with our little boy and the other kids. What a coward I am! What would he do all alone? And Johnny—he needs me even if I'm not much of a mother. If I just knew what to do! If I could just be patient like other mothers.

This statement by the patient is an excellent example of a fairly predictable process: if negative feelings are consistently accepted, the patient tends to move from a totally negative position toward ambivalence or a partially positive one.

NURSE:
You get angry with yourself when you are impatient with your children.

The nurse has made several responses that have helped identify the patient's feelings. The patient can now look at the feelings herself with less turmoil. Further, she sees that the nurse understands and does not blame her for having such feelings.

PATIENT:
I do get angry at the other children, but I don't feel so bad when I jump on them.

NURSE:
It's more difficult with John, because he has special problems.

PATIENT:
Yes, I feel so helpless with John. I guess if I knew how to work with him better I wouldn't be so impatient.

The purpose of exploring and examining feelings is to help the patient see how they relate to her problem. Mrs. Carson has identified her problem as being an inadequate mother to a child with special needs.

NURSE:
There is a social worker on our staff who works with children who have special problems. She might be helpful to you and John, and if you feel you would like to talk with her, it can be arranged.

Note that the nurse has not offered recommendations on the basis of an early inference of what she suspected the problem might be, but only after the patient has been helped to identify her problem. In addition, she informed the patient of a relevant resource, giving her the opportunity for choice rather than urging a particular course of action.

PATIENT:
Yes, I would. I used to talk with John's teacher, and that helped a lot, but since he hasn't been in school, I haven't seen her. We must get him back in school soon.

We will have to borrow money for the operation; that is why his schooling has to wait. I wish there were some way to pay for both at the same time.

NURSE:
The social worker I mentioned also has some experience in helping with financial problems.

PATIENT:
Could my husband and I both talk to her before I have the operation? I would want him to see her with me.

As she was helped to express and clarify her feelings, Mrs. Carson replaced her desperate thoughts of death as a solution with a more constructive approach. She began to consider making plans for the care of her child and to think about working out her financial problems.

This interchange illustrates another axiom of interviewing. When upset and confused, the patient cannot explain problems or express feelings logically or sequentially. The story is apt to be told in a piece-meal, jumbled fashion. The interviewer need not "push" a plan or answer. Through the use of the principles already discussed—listening, accepting, offering appropriate information—solutions begin to emerge.

## VALID REASSURANCE

The foregoing makes it apparent that conventional verbal reassurance is of little value. Yet all of us have known at one time or another the sense of relief that comes from feeling really reassured. What means accomplish this end?

### Respect for the Patient

Individuals experience reassurance when, under stress, they find themselves listened to, respected, and understood rather than overwhelmed with advice or empty words of consolation. They feel "safe" enough to explore and identify their own feelings and problems. With timely information they usually can develop appropriate resources for managing their difficulties. The interaction between Mrs. Carson and the nurse is illustrative. One senses that Mrs. Carson experienced true reassurance from the nurse's genuine interest, her willingness to listen, and, perhaps most, from the deep respect she demonstrated in her attention to a confused and desperate woman.

## Giving Correct Information

On the day after a hemorrhoidectomy, a patient had the urge to urinate but could not start his stream. He became extremely anxious and fantasied that a surgical error had been committed. Awakening from a nightmare in which he dreamed of having to be catheterized, he rang for the nurse and demanded an explanation, threatening to sue the hospital and surgeons. The nurse explained that his inability to start the urinary stream was a typical postoperative symptom after rectal surgery, and that additional sitz baths would help. The patient distrusted this information, until he tested the nurse's recommendation. Had he been given this information before surgery, or as soon after as possible, he would have been spared much anxiety.

A patient can feel genuinely reassured when given correct information at the time it is needed by a trusted person. Two aspects of this principle must be emphasized: (1) the information must be authentic, and (2) it must be given by someone in whom the patient has confidence. To tell a patient, for example, that he or she will definitely feel better after taking a pill would not meet these requirements. It is well known that medications do not always have the desired effect. Similarly, information would not be reassuring, no matter how authentic, if given by a professional person who previously had been less than honest with the patient.

## Limit Setting

In this discussion, our theses have tended to emphasize the "permissive" aspects of the professional relationship. As in all aspects of living, however, limits to self-expression and patient behavior must be recognized. Reasonable restrictions are not only necessary, but helpful to all of us in regulating our lives and our relations to others.

The positive value of appropriate limits lies in the fact that they provide structure in otherwise amorphous situations and hence reduce anxiety. A teenager is probably more comfortable knowing that permission to drive the family car will be withdrawn if he or she is involved in careless traffic violations. It will be reassuring to a hospitalized patient when the physician or nurse enforces a limit preventing behavior that may damage her- or himself or others. It is also reassuring to a patient to be oriented to hospital rules, provided they are reasonable and fairly enforced.

In Chapters 2 and 4, we have pointed out that a patient may wish to become socially involved with the physician or nurse. Health professionals will wisely limit such contacts by explaining that they can be most useful in their professional capacity and therefore do not become involved in the social life of patients. The patient will find it reassuring that health workers maintain this type of relationship, since it is easier to discuss personal matters with someone with whom one is not socially involved. The patient will find the relationship to the health professionals stable and predictable.

## Referral

In Chapter 9 in the discussion of referrals, we will comment on the care that must be taken when a patient needs the services of specialists or another member of the health team. A referral can constitute a break in the physician–patient relationship. Patients may wonder if the physician either is rejecting them or is not competent to handle the problem. However, a referral to a specially trained person can be reassuring rather than confusing or rejecting if the services of others are skillfully interpreted and if the referring physician remains, whenever possible, in charge of the case.

## Physical Presence of a Trusted Person

At times a patient may be so terrified, eg, just prior to surgery or during labor, that verbal interchange is almost impossible. These circumstances are most common with children, sometimes even during routine examinations. In such temporary crises, the patient may be reassured by the physical presence of someone trusted, whose calm holding of a hand, perhaps with no words spoken, or whose quiet statement that he or she will stand by, communicates that the patient has not been abandoned. When terror subsides, the patient may be more able to talk about and understand the exaggerated nature of these feelings. The reassuring experience perhaps serves to reduce fear on the next occasion when similar procedures are necessary.

## SUMMARY

The reassuring response has been defined as one in which the health professional, in effect, denies that the patient has a problem and suggests that the patient need not feel this way. A patient is not likely to reveal anxieties after having been told that they do not or should not exist. Self-confidence develops from within the patient, not from without. Consequently, the patient can achieve assurance from having an opportunity to explore and understand his or her own feelings.

By exposing feelings the patient indicates a desire to discuss them. A conventionally reassuring response communicates to the patient that health professionals would prefer not to discuss such matters, often because the feelings expressed are upsetting to them. For this reason, it has been stated that a reassuring response serves to protect the feelings of the members of the health team and not those of the patient.

Health professionals sometimes rely on spurious methods to ease or quiet the patient. Falsification merely postpones discovery of the truth. When the truth is learned, the situation will become more difficult to handle. This awkward circumstance would not have arisen if the health worker had responded honestly to the feelings in the first place.

Introducing irrelevant material to distract the patient from painful areas interferes with modification of feelings, whereas dealing with feelings and attitudes facilitates modification. Consequently health professionals must sensitize themselves to the immediate feelings and not divert the patient by changing the subject or by introducing irrelevant topics.

Professional persons' most extreme tactic for protecting themselves from unpleasant situations or discussions is avoidance—staying away from the patient.

Genuine reassurance comes from a demonstration of respect for the patient. An understanding relationship helps the patient to identify feelings and problems and develop appropriate resources for managing them.

A patient can also experience reassurance when given correct information at the time it is needed, by a trusted person.

Reasonable limit setting can create reassurance by providing structure to a situation and hence reducing anxiety.

Referral to a specially trained person can be reassuring if the services of others are skillfully interpreted to the patient and if the referring physician remains, whenever possible, in charge of the case.

The quiet presence of a trusted person in times of overwhelming fear, eg, before surgery or during delivery, can provide real reassurance.

## REFERENCES

1. Glaser BG, Strauss AL: Awareness of Dying. Chicago, Aldine, 1965
2. Gregg D: Reassurance. Am J Nurs 55:171, 1955
3. Wolberg LR: The Technique of Psychotherapy, 2nd ed. New York, Grune & Stratton, 1967

# chapter 6

# The Probing Response

If one listens to beginning students of interviewing, one has the distinct impression that they consider the question their basic tool. We know, however, that a patient who has responded to a series of questions actually develops an expectation that the interviewer will be able to offer an answer or solution to the problem. The probing (questioning) response then becomes an extension of the evaluative, advice-giving techniques, and has the same limitations already discussed in Chapter 3.

Probing, or questioning, tends to follow certain patterns. One is the irrelevant question, inappropriate to the material. Another is the stereotyped series of questions often used in taking a patient's history. However, there are other, more productive methods of obtaining specific information, necessary for diagnosis and treatment. These will be discussed later.

## ASKING IRRELEVANT QUESTIONS

Physicians and nurses frequently ask questions about the specific time and place of events in order to satisfy their own curiosity, often at an inappropriate time for the patient, for no apparent reason. For example, a man is describing intensely his wife's "back-seat driving," which led him to divert his attention from the road and caused the accident that brought him to the hospital two days before. This expression of anger is interrupted by the nurse who asks, "Did the accident happen at night or during the day?" and then "Was it on a two-lane highway?" These questions have little to do with the patient's present troubles. The accident has happened; whether it occurred by day or at night, on a two-lane highway or on a freeway is less important at this time than the patient's need to express his tension about the events that led to the accident. Questions of time, place, speed, injuries to others, etc, are appropriate for the sheriff investigating the accident. For the nurse or physician, the answers to such questions, which eventually may be given spontaneously, are secondary.

The patient will give all the information we are seeking—and more—if he or she can be helped to tell the story in his or her own way and in an open manner. Although the information may not emerge in precise order, neither will important information be deleted. It should be emphasized that questions can guide the flow of but cannot produce information.

As noted previously, unless health professionals have given special attention to or have had specific training in interviewing, they are apt to take their cues for verbal interaction from their personal and social experience. In a social situation silence can become embarrassing and uncomfortable. To avoid this discomfort we are prone to ask questions of those with whom we are interacting. In professional situations such questions frequently tend to be irrelevant or to open areas the interviewer is unprepared to handle.

For example, a nurse submitted the following incident to us for review:

Mr. M, an elderly cardiac patient, was sitting in his chair as I made his bed. Usually talkative, this morning he remained silent.

NURSE:
Are you married, Mr. M? (I remembered seeing on his chart that he was, so I felt it was a safe, normal question.)

Apparently the nurse could not tolerate the patient's silence and felt compelled to ask a "safe, normal question."
She had several more appropriate alternatives. She could have respected the patient's wish to be silent. Or she might have reflected the patient's silence with a comment such as: "You're unusually quiet this morning."

MR. M:
I was until my wife died last month.
(Tears came to his eyes.)

Mr. M could have made a "yes" or "no" response. The fact that he mentions his wife's recent death suggests that he may wish to discuss his loss.

NURSE:
Oh, I'm sorry. I wouldn't have brought it up—er—a—. (I was completely floored, as I was not expecting this answer.)

The nurse, expecting to start a pleasant social conversation, is unprepared for Mr. M's emotional response.

Again, the nurse had a more appropriate alternative. She could have shifted from her expectation of a bit of social chit-chat to recognizing the patient's feelings, perhaps with a comment such as "That must have been a terrible loss for you," or "It's still hard to live with, isn't it?"

MR. M:
I've never seen a person suffer as she did, especially those last three months.
(Tears continue to flow.)

The patient indicates that he wishes to continue talking, in spite of the nurse's desire to close the topic she inadvertently has opened.

NURSE:
That's a shame. (Flustered again. Several answers flickered through my mind, all of them inadequate. So I uttered a platitude and left the room.)

The nurse might have responded more appropriately with something in the nature of, "It must have been awful for you to see her suffer so."

In this incident a casual question opened a serious emotional wound and created a tense situation from which the nurse retreated. The patient might well wonder why such a question was asked, if his honest answer brought no more than "a platitude." The nurse, after blundering into this painful area, could have redeemed the situation by allowing this patient the healing experience of expressing his mourning.

We see a similar outcome in the following interaction between a medical student and a patient. During evening rounds, Mr. P, age 60, spoke of his wife.

MR. P:
You can tell she's a good woman just by looking at her. (Obvious pride was evident in his voice and expression.)

MEDICAL STUDENT:
Do you have any children? (Question was asked simply for conversation.)

This response is puzzling. In his parenthetic remark following the patient's opening statement, the student recognizes the patient's pride. Rather than indicating his recognition, however, he asks a question "simply for conversation."

MR. P:
Not by her. I was married before and have five children by my first wife. (Patient lowered his eyes, spoke more softly than before. He seemed to become tense.)

MEDICAL STUDENT:
Oh, how nice!

The student is aware of the patient's tension. Yet he replies with the social platitude that is expected when one's children are mentioned.

MR. P:
No, it wasn't! She ran around and never bothered about fixing meals for the kids or anything. What would *you* think of a woman like that? (He looked at me very intensely as he asked this question.)

MEDICAL STUDENT:
Oh—I don't know. Uh—I have to finish my rounds. I'll see you tomorrow. (I'm sure my face red-

In his confusion, the student could only escape. Had he felt less embarrassed, he might have re-

dened as I left the room.)                    covered by a comment to the effect,
                                              "The way she acted certainly was
                                              hard on you."

    In these two incidents the message to the patient was that the
interviewer preferred to avoid expressions of feelings, in spite of the
fact that the interviewer's question elicited them in the first place. In
each of these incidents the opportunity to allow emotional relief was
missed. While not every casual encounter can become a therapeutic
experience, professional personnel need to be alert to the meaning of
even brief, everyday interactions with patients.

## HISTORY TAKING

History taking has a unique importance in medical practice. It can
clarify diagnosis and give direction to treatment plans. It also presents
special problems and requires skillful procedure.
    In taking an initial history on a patient, the interviewer has the
choice of using: (1) a prepared or stereotyped series of direct questions,
often asked in a rapid-fire manner described as the "Mr. District Attorney" approach, or (2) an open interview in which the interviewer's
task is to help the patient talk freely with appropriate and necessary
guidance.

### The Direct-Question Approach

Especially in an initial or early contact with a patient, the technique of
asking a series of short, rapid questions has serious limitations. Such
interviews prevent the patient from telling his or her own story. They
interrupt a patient's sequence of thought—if a sequence of thought has
been allowed to develop. They may divert the patient into discussing
unimportant and irrelevant matters. The following is a condensation
of such an interview, characterized by overly specific and staccato
questions:

PHYSICIAN:
What symptoms bring you here?

PATIENT:
Last night I woke up with a terrific pain in my stomach—right here
(points).

PHYSICIAN:
Ever had it before?

PATIENT:
No, not that bad.

PHYSICIAN:
You had it before, but not so bad?

PATIENT:
Not really, I've had mild stomach aches before but nothing like this.

PHYSICIAN:
Any other complaints?

PATIENT:
No sir.

PHYSICIAN:
Ever had diabetes, tuberculosis, kidney, or liver disease?

PATIENT:
No.

PHYSICIAN:
Ever had any operations?

PATIENT:
Just my tonsils taken out.

PHYSICIAN:
How long ago?

PATIENT:
I must have been about five.

PHYSICIAN:
Are you on any special diet?

PATIENT:
No, but I am trying to watch my weight.

PHYSICIAN:
You overweight?

PATIENT:
I don't know.

PHYSICIAN:
Well, we'll weigh you later. Do you smoke?

PATIENT:
Yes. About a pack a day.

PHYSICIAN:
How about alcohol?

PATIENT:
Just an occasional drink at a party. I might have a beer after work
sometimes.

PHYSICIAN:
Ever been drunk?

PATIENT:
No sir.

PHYSICIAN:
Are you taking medication for anything?

PATIENT:
No. I've been pretty healthy all my life. Just this thing last night
scared me.

PHYSICIAN:
Is your father living and well?

PATIENT:
Yes.

PHYSICIAN:
Mother too?

PATIENT:
Yes.

PHYSICIAN:
Any bothers or sisters?

PATIENT:
One sister.

PHYSICIAN:
How's her health?

PATIENT:
Fine, as far as I know.

PHYSICIAN:
As far as you know?

PATIENT:
Well, she's living out of town. We hear from her regularly and she's never mentioned any serious illness.

PHYSICIAN:
I see. What does your father do?

PATIENT:
He's a fireman.

PHYSICIAN:
O.K. Now go in there, strip to the waist, and we'll see what we can find.


This interview revealed information of an almost statistical nature. These data could have been obtained as well if the patient had completed a routine form in the waiting room or the hospital admission office. More seriously, by using an interviewing method that limited the patient's responses, the physician may have missed important information, perhaps more relevant than the occupation of his father. The question - answer format may also have implied that the physician has so specialized and mysterious a knowledge of what is important and relevant that the patient is likely to refrain from any spontaneous comment and respond only to specific questions. This observation led Balint[1] to conclude that " . . . if you ask questions, you get answers— and hardly anything else" (p. 133). Parenthetically, it should be noted that in some situations, such as a brief emergency-room interview with a patient in severe pain, the direct-question approach is quite appropriate, so long as the questions are clearly relevant.

Sheppe and Stevenson[4] have pointed out that a successful medical interview has three main goals: (1) to establish a positive physician-patient relationship; (2) to elicit information about the patient's condition; and (3) to permit observation of the patient's behavior. A series of direct questions and answers may accomplish the second goal, but the other two purposes of the interview are inevitably neglected. It has been suggested repeatedly that encouraging the patient to talk freely by an empathic listener promotes the relationship, and the patient who senses a friendly relationship with health professionals will be more cooperative in treatment. The patient is also more likely to demonstrate typical behavior when feeling comfortable and at ease. The physician and nurse will have valuable information as to what to expect in future contacts. It becomes apparent, then, that the three tasks of the interview can be achieved simultaneously.

## The Open Interview

In an open interview a broad subject is offered at first. Usually it begins with a discussion of the presenting complaint. However, all interviews need not start with, "What is your symptom?" since the discussion is then confined to too narrow a range. It is more productive to ask, "What is it you wanted to see me about?" or "When you phoned for an appointment, you said you felt run down. Could you tell me more about that?" Such questions open rather than limit the area of discussion.

When the patient has begun to talk, the explanation should be allowed to continue, preferably without interruption. Pauses or points of hesitation should not be used to change course but as an opportunity to express interest, offer encouragement, or ask for clarification. Of major interest will be the manner in which the patient formulates the complaints, how concerned he or she is about them, and whether they are related to other life events. The interviewer should also be alert to the sequence and order of events described. Quite frequently patients will describe one symptom and, if not interrupted, will mention other symptoms in the context of recent stresses in their lives.

The following is the early phase of an open interview:

PHYSICIAN:
I wonder if you could tell me something about why you've come to see me?

PATIENT:
Well, like I told your nurse—you know, when I called for an appointment—I've been having these headaches. They started about a month

ago and they've been getting worse—to the point where I'm embarrassed about going to work. When one comes on at work, I have to hide, the pain's so bad. Last week I stayed home and called in sick every day. But I can't go on doing that.

PHYSICIAN:
Uh-hm.

PATIENT:
You see, I'm the head seamstress at _____ (a women's dress shop). The spring season is on us, and we're already behind in our alteration work. And we'll just have to get the Easter outfits ready on time. I can just hear the customers complaining.

PHYSICIAN:
Yes, I can understand that.

PATIENT:
I suppose I might as well tell you, doctor, I've been worried about a brain tumor. My father died of a brain tumor just about a year ago this month. And then Mother moved in with us—with my husband and me. We'd only been married three months when he passed away. My mother's pretty bossy, and it didn't help a new marriage to have her so close. Then last month I discovered I was pregnant. I've been reading some books on the subject—you know, about how an expectant mother should be calm and relaxed during pregnancy. It could affect the child, you know. And I'd like to be relaxed. But how can I be with my mother nagging that we're not ready to have a child—uh, and now these awful headaches. And my husband still has another year of college—he's going to be an accountant. And if I don't get back to work soon, what will we use for money?

PHYSICIAN:
I can see you feel pretty desperate right now.

PATIENT:
You can say that again, doctor. You know, I've always looked forward to pregnancy. But not I don't know. The headaches started just after I found out I was pregnant. And I've been wondering whether the two are connected in some way. Do I really want a child now, before Frank—that's my husband—can support us? Maybe my mother's right.

PHYSICIAN:
You see some connection between your pregnancy and your headaches?

PATIENT:
I've certainly thought about it. I've had minor headaches before. Just
the usual kind that would go away after a few aspirin tablets. But
aspirin won't touch these. And after a month of them, I'm desperate.

PHYSICIAN:
Uh-hm.

PATIENT:
I'm even beginning to wonder if I'm worried about a brain tumor or
*hoping* it's a brain tumor. If it is a tumor, I wouldn't have to face up to
the pregnancy. Oh, God, but I'm confused!


Headaches are certainly a frequent presenting complaint. After
this patient's initial mention of headaches, the physician had several
choices. He might have attempted to localize the pain and concentrate
on diagnosing the headaches. He might have inquired about other
symptoms or begun taking a history. The significant circumstances of
her life situation, which seem to have a direct relationship to the
headaches, would not have been revealed.

It should be noted how much important data the physician has
been given without asking more than the opening question: the duration of the patient's symptoms, her occupation, her husband's status
and vocational goal, information about the father's death, her attitudes toward the mother, the time of her marriage, and her present
pregnant state. Perhaps more important, the possible connection between her symptoms and her pregnancy has been suggested. The physician can now formulate several potentially fruitful hypotheses
worthy of further diagnostic exploration. Are the headaches associated
with anger toward the mother as well as anxiety about the pregnancy?
Since the father died "just about a year ago this month," could the
symptoms represent an anniversary reaction to that event?

Not every patient will be as free in communicating as this one.
When patients seem to want to continue talking but appear hesitant or
blocked, a certain kind of statement can help them continue. For example, the physician or nurse might say, "I'm not quite sure I understand.
Can you explain that a little more?" or, "I can see that this is something important for you. Go on, if you'd like." These methods encourage patients to enlarge on matters that they themselves have introduced without making them feel that the interviewer is prying.

At times the patient will appear to have reached a dead end with a
comment such as, "That's about all I can say about it," or "I don't know
what else to say." In a situation such as this, the interviewer can

inquire about a topic discussed earlier in the interview, eg, "You were telling me that your mother was bossy. Does that have something to do with this problem you've been talking about?" This approach will keep the interview focused on the patient's concerns and is more appropriate than introducing a new topic.

## OBTAINING SPECIFIC INFORMATION

Even in the most successful open interview, there will be areas about which more information is needed. Direct questions will have to be asked. However, there is a vast difference between an interview limited entirely to a brief question, "Yes" or "No" answer session, and one in which questions are asked after the patient has been permitted to give his or her own account of matters. In the latter case the question serves as clarification rather than interference.

Several principles are helpful in the use of direct questions:

1. The sequence of questions should progress from the general to the specific.
2. The questions should be worded to elicit longer answers than "yes" or "no" responses.
3. The questions should be worded to avoid bias.
4. "Why" questions usually should not be asked.

### Progression from the General to the Specific

The open interview is begun with the most general kind of question, such as "What led to your coming to see me?" The patient then has a free range with no predetermined focus.

In asking questions, the physician might start with a relatively broad question, followed by progressively more detailed questions. This process is frequently referred to as *narrowing* and is particularly useful for eliciting important and spontaneous patient attitudes. For example, following the beginning of the open interview above, the first question might have been "You say you think your pregnancy has something to do with the headaches. Can you tell me why you feel that way?" Possibly the patient might then give further expression to her dread of having a child. The physician could continue with a question or questions clarifying which factors in the patient's life give rise to the dread—financial problems, her mother's disapproval, her husband's disappointment that he may not be able to continue his education, perhaps even her own basic reluctance to assume this responsibility. As the discussion becomes more specific, the ground is laid for later consideration of possible solutions to each problem. (It goes without saying that the physician will also make appropriate medical investigation of the headaches.)

## Avoiding Questions That Elicit "Yes" or "No" Answers

Even when specific questions must be asked, the interviewer's aim should be to help the patient continue to talk freely. Therefore questions should be worded to elicit more than a one-word response. When a question passes the initiative to the patient, it is known as an *open* question. A *closed* question is one that the patient can answer with "yes" or "no." There are clear advantages to asking "What was the pain like?" rather than "Was the pain sharp?", "How was your last pregnancy?" instead of "Did you have much nausea during your last pregnancy?"

## Avoiding Interviewer Bias

The patient's responses in any interview depend largely on the wording of the questions. There are several ways in which interviewers inadvertently bias the patient's answers.

### Question Loading

"Loading" refers to asking a question in a manner that makes it more likely for the patient to give one answer rather than another. For example, during a physical examination, if the physician says, "This area isn't very painful, is it?" the patient may well assume that the physician expects a "no," and may be reluctant to contradict the physician. Although the patient's reply may appear to confirm the physician's hypothesis, the physician cannot be certain that it is not his or her powers of suggestion that have been confirmed.

Another variety of loaded question occurs when we use words that are highly charged emotionally. In the field of medicine, "cancer" is certainly such a word. Evidence of a connection between smoking and lung malignancy has led to a certain stigma associated with the use of tobacco. Patients who are defensive about smoking may answer less than truthfully questions such as: "How long have you smoked?" "How many cigarettes do you smoke each day?"

The effects of loaded questions are especially serious in a medical setting. Patients are likely to feel dependent on and subordinate to the nurse or physician. Consequently they may be highly sensitive to the interviewer's language and more apt to give a response they think is expected. Answers can then lead to a misunderstanding of the complaints and consequent diagnostic errors. Loaded questions may also seriously interfere with the physician-patient and nurse-patient relationships. The patient may feel inadvertently "trapped" into giving incorrect answers and, aware of the serious results of misinformation, feel guilty, concerned, and angry.

### Double-Barreled Questions
Biased answers are likely to follow double-barreled questions—in which only one answer can be given to two or more questions. For example:

PHYSICIAN:
Do you take pills and follow a diet for your nausea?

PATIENT:
Yes.

PHYSICIAN:
Is your nausea controlled and your general health good?

PATIENT:
Yes.

Actually the physician has asked two successive double-barreled questions so that the patient's "yes" replies are highly ambiguous. If each of the four questions has bearing on the diagnosis and treatment, the physician will have to backtrack and repeat them separately. The question-and-answer technique is often justified as time-saving, but in this instance the physician has wasted his own and the patient's time. Relatively simple, straightforward points of fact may now require complicated clarification.

### Vocabulary Level of Questions
Health professionals do not share a common vocabulary with most patients. A humorous illustration of this disparity was reported to us by a student nurse. In preparing a patient for electroshock therapy, she asked, "Do you have dentures?" The patient replied, "No, I have schizophrenia." When a patient responds to the question, "Has there been much tussis with your chest pains?" the "yes" or "no" may be

covering the patient's embarrassment about not knowing what *tussis* is. It is obviously important to use language that is clear to the patient. However, the solution is not always simplified language. The interviewer can gauge from the first interaction with the patient what level of communication is appropriate. For a patient with a relatively good vocabulary, oversimplification may mean that his or her intellectual capacity is being underestimated. The relationship between patient and interviewer will be strengthened when the health professional can tailor language to the vocabulary level of the patient.

Almost always care should be taken to avoid medical jargon. A study of 800 tape-recorded interviews conducted in the outpatient department of the Los Angeles Children's Hospital[3] indicated that physicians were using terms incomprehensible even to lay persons of high intelligence. For example, mothers who were questioned indicated that they had no knowledge of terms such as nares, peristalsis, or Coombs' titre. One mother thought that "lumbar puncture" was an operation to drain the lungs. "Incubation period" was interpreted to mean the length of time the child should stay in bed. There was no indication that hospitalization was implied when her child was to be "admitted for a workup." Nor was surgery expected when the physician stated that he or she would have to explore.

### Misinterpretation of Patient Response

Another source of bias may occur when a patient's response is interpreted in keeping with the interviewer's own expectations. The physician may ask, "Have you had the usual childhood diseases?" An affirmative reply may mean to the physician that the patient has had mumps, measles, and whooping cough. For the patient, "usual" may have meant rheumatic fever, too. If another opportunity does not present itself to add this bit of information, the physician will have lost an important diagnostic clue.

## Avoiding "Why" Questions

Benjamin[2] makes a strong case for avoiding questions asking "why." "Why" may have two meanings. It can be a way of seeking information or, more often, it can imply disapproval. A mother who says to her child, "Why must you be so messy at the table?" is not seeking information; she is critizing the child's manners. Sensing the meaning of "why" questions, children learn to defend themselves by answering, "Because." Eventually, children learn to use "why" in this manner themselves. A child who asks, "Why do I have to take piano lessons?" is not expecting an explanation, but is saying, "I don't want to take piano lessons." Having thus learned the negative meaning of "why" over the years, the patient in the interview situation may react to it as an indication of disapproval and respond defensively.

There are further reasons for avoiding "why" questions. Frequently persons will give merely socially acceptable answers when the "why" of their own behavior is not quite clear to them, perhaps based on only dimly perceived motivation. Thus, health professionals, when asked why they chose their particular careers, are likely to speak of a wish to help people, rather than a desire for status and high income. Some patients may well know the "why" of their behavior but be quite unwilling to reveal it. For example, a geriatric man, when asked why he has not taken his medication, may say that he forgot and complain about his memory when in reality he has not found the medication helpful but is fearful of saying so. Health professionals are more likely to be told the truth if they maintain a consistently accepting and empathic relationship, rather than asking the threatening "why."

## SUMMARY

A probing response implies that the patient might profitably give more information so that the interviewer may be able to offer an answer or solution to the problem. When used in this manner, the probing response becomes an extension of the evaluative, advice-giving techniques and has the same limitations.

To avoid the discomfort of silence in a verbal interchange, health professionals may ask personal questions of their patients. Frequently such questions open areas that the interviewer is unprepared to handle. When the health worker attempts to avoid the feelings the questions have precipitated, the patient is left wondering why the questions were asked in the first place.

The use of a series of short, rapid questions in taking a history prevents the patient from telling his or her own story. Such questions interrupt a patient's sequence of thought and may sidetrack the discussion into unimportant and irrelevant matters. In certain emergency situations, direct questions may be appropriate.

Physicians and nurses frequently ask questions about the specific time and place of events for no apparent reason. These questions not only divert the patient but may be irrelevant.

Questions can guide the flow of information but cannot produce it.

Patients will give all the information we are seeking if they can be helped to tell their story their own way and in an open manner.

The goals of a successful interview in a medical setting are to establish a positive relationship, to elicit information about the patient's condition, and to permit observation of behavior. These tasks can be achieved simultaneously by permitting the patient to talk freely in the presence of an empathic listener.

In an open interview the patient is offered a broad subject to discuss at first. Of major interest will be the manner in which the patient formulates complaints, how concerned the patient is about them, and whether they are related to other life events. A patient who seems to want to continue talking, but appears hesitant or blocked, may be offered leads that encourage elaboration on matters he or she has introduced.

Even in the most successful open interview there will be areas about which more information will be needed. Direct questions will have to be asked. Several principles should be followed in the use of direct questions. The sequence of questions should proceed from the general to the specific. Questions should be worded in a manner that elicits more than a one-word response. An open question is one that passes the initiative to the patient, whereas a closed question is one that the patient can answer with a "yes" or "no." Questions should be worded to avoid biasing the patient's answers. A loaded question is one that is asked in a manner that makes it easier, although not necessarily more accurate, for the patient to give one answer rather than another. Biased answers can also be elicited by asking a double-barreled question in which one answer serves for two or more questions. The vocabulary level of questions may also produce inaccurate answers. The use of language that is not clear to the patient interferes with communication, since the patient is being asked to respond to something that is not understood. For a patient with a relatively good vocabulary, oversimplification may mean that his or her intellectual capacity is being underestimated. Since language is the single most important ingredient in communication, health professionals must learn to tailor their vocabularies to the individual patient. However, with all patients medical jargon and "why" questions should be avoided.

# REFERENCES

1. Balint M: The Doctor, His Patient and the Illness. New York, International Universities Press, 1957

2. Benjamin A: The Helping Interview, 2nd ed. Boston, Houghton Mifflin, 1974
3. Korsch BM, Negrete VF: Doctor-patient communication. Sci Am 227:66, 1972
4. Sheppe WM Jr, Stevenson I: Techniques of interviewing. In Lief HI, Lief FV, Lief NR (eds): The Psychological Basis of Medical Practice. New York, Hoeber, 1963

# chapter 7

# The Understanding Response

*"First of all," he said, "if you can learn a simple trick, Scout, you'll get along a lot better with all kinds of folks. You never really understand a person until you consider things from his point of view —"*
    *"Sir?"*
    *"—until you climb into his skin and walk around in it."*[7]

This quotation from *To Kill A Mockingbird* captures the essence of the understanding response. It will be recalled that the understanding response is described as one in which the health professional attempts to comprehend the patient's point of view and, by communicating that comprehension, helps the patient clarify and cope with the problem. By now the reader is quite familiar with this concept since in Chapters 3 through 6 we have contrasted the understanding response with each of the other four categories.

It is a truism that people tend to relate best to those who understand them. In the usual relationships and experiences of daily life, it is readily observed that we feel better and perform better when we sense that we are understood. The explanation for this common phenomenon is that understanding serves to diminish fear and anxiety. When free, or relatively free, of these constrictions, we are more likely to behave constructively and effectively.

Understanding implies acceptance. Acceptance, which does *not* imply agreement or approval, escapes precise definition as a word and as a concept, although it is in common use, particularly in interviewing and all forms of counseling. *Acceptance* is more easily described in its implications and effects. It can be equated with a deep respect, which goes hand in hand with a profound recognition that "the other" is always different, never perfect, a compendium of positive and negative, mature and immature forces. For most of life, change and growth are possible. If one's potential is to be realized, however, favorable circumstances are necessary to foster maturation. "The seed cannot flourish in hostile soil." *Favorable* in this context does not mean *advantaged* or *problem-free*. It does mean opportunity to develop and use those inner resources that encourage problem solving and effective living. Good relationships can offer that opportunity.

If understanding and acceptance, good relationships and opportunity, are fundamental in the ordinary circumstances of life, how much more important are they under conditions of illness and stress. We have already emphasized in previous chapters and in case examples the significant role health professionals potentially play in their relationships with patients. We wish to pursue this theme now by examining the way in which the quality of understanding can be developed and used. For many professionals, particularly students, a consciousness of their role can be threatening and anxiety-producing, as though too great a responsibility has been thrust upon them. Developing the capacity to understand, to accept, to relate may seem too amorphous and too overwhelming a task. Yet these qualities are neither innate nor mysterious. They are akin to skills in interviewing (Chapter 2), and they too can almost always be taught and learned.

## CAN ONE LEARN TO ESTABLISH TRUSTING RELATIONSHIPS WITH OTHERS?

Our own optimism is matched by a prevalent skepticism that the skills required for understanding relationships with patients can become the subject matter for professional teaching. For example, in a study by Shields,[10] individuals associated with schools of nursing, public health agencies, and other nursing groups were asked by questionnaire to indicate whether they thought a basic nursing curriculum should provide learning experiences intended to develop certain qualities or abilities. One such quality was described as " . . . a belief in the essential worth of every human being . . . and the importance of communicating this belief by attitudes and actions" (p. 12).

Although a large percentage of those who replied to the questionnaire felt that this was an important skill, some of the comments of the respondents reflected a doubt that such a quality could be taught:

A person either has or hasn't this quality. Shouldn't be a nurse if she hasn't it. Can't be taught (supervisor of a visiting nurse association).

This comes with maturity and cannot be taught (private duty nurse).
Criminals too? (private duty nurse)
Idealistic. Impossible. *No one* can really believe in the essential worth of every human being (director of a school).
Belongs in family teaching, not nursing education (p. 12).

## Research on Nurses' Attitudes

In view of this skepticism, it appeared worthwhile to investigate empirically whether nurse-patient relationships based upon the concepts proposed in this book could be taught successfully. A study was devised[4] to test the hypothesis that nurses' skills and attitudes in interpersonal relationships can be modified in a positive way when nurses understand the nature of the techniques they use, the attitudes such techniques express or implement, and the feelings they generate in patients.

Thirty nurses participated in ten two-hour weekly sessions with the senior investigator. The course began with a presentation of the basic techniques nurses use in responding to patients, a discussion of the attitudes these techniques express, and a discussion of how the patient might react to each of these techniques. For the remainder of the course, nurses brought to class incidents from their interactions with patients. Discussion of these incidents centered on the feelings the patient was expressing and how the nurse might best respond.

Before and after this training, the nurses who participated, as well as a comparable group of nurses who did not participate, took the Nurse–Patient Situation Test. This test was made up of 35 typical nurse-patient incidents in which a patient's comment to the nurse and five possible responses were presented. In each test item, the possible nurse responses included an evaluative response, a hostile response, a reassuring response, a probing response, and an understanding response. The nurses were asked to select the one they thought was the most appropriate.

Before training, less than 15 percent of the nurse responses were understanding; after training, 80 percent were in the understanding category. Those who did not participate in the training showed no significant change when the test was taken a second time.

The question may well be asked whether the Nurse–Patient Situation Test is not a direct measure of the content of the course, and therefore may not reflect a basic change in underlying attitudes. Consequently other independent measures (tests) of attitude change were included in the experimental situation.

One test was the F-Scale.[1] This scale measures attitudes on a continuum, ranging from authoritarian to democratic or equalitarian. It was found that, although there were no differences between the groups on the pretest, on the post-test the group exposed to training, but not the control group, showed a significant shift toward more democratic attitudes.

A second independent measure of change consisted of reading to both groups a lengthy case history. The items in the history could be classified as physical (temperature, blood pressure, diagnoses, laboratory procedures, medications, and so forth) and psychosocial (patient's ward behavior, degree of dependency, employment history, relations with hospital personnel and visitors, and so forth). Immediately after the history had been read, the subjects were asked to write down everything they remembered. Again it was found that there were no differences between the groups on the pretest in the ratio of psychosocial to physical items. However, on the post-test, the group that had received training showed a higher degree of sensitivity to the psychosocial factors in the history. In addition, supervisors of the nurses who participated in the training program reported that these students were dealing more effectively with their patients.

## Research on Medical Students' Attitudes

A variation of the above study[3] was undertaken with medical students. The Nurse–Patient Situation Test was converted to the Physician–Patient Situation Test and administered to 102 first-year medical students on the first and last days of a 12-week course in the Physician–Patient Relationship. The emphasis in the course was on supervised bedside interviewing of patients (see Preface for a more detailed description of the course). At the completion of the course, there was a highly significant increase in the number of understanding responses selected on the test. However, to determine whether they were actually using more understanding responses, a sample of 16 students was requested to record their first and last interviews of the semester. The tapes were rated by a group of five faculty judges who did not know the students' identities or whether they were listening to a first or last interview. Again it was found that the final interviews showed a significant increase in the use of understanding responses.

In a related study[5] 100 first-year and 100 second-year medical students took a test of "clinical judgment," devised by Ashby et al.[2]

This test measures the willingness and/or ability to accept what a patient has to say without feeling a need to evaluate, judge, or criticize. The test consists of statements of beliefs, opinions, and values made by unidentified individuals. These items represent viewpoints deviant from those of medical students, but not so deviant as to warrant their being labeled pathologic. For example, the following statement of opinion is one item: "You get a wild kid—the only way to handle him is to break him. Otherwise he'll end up a crook or something." The students' task was to classify the statements as having been made by an adjusted or maladjusted individual. It was reasoned that those who classified fewer items as maladjusted would be those who would most readily accept the values of others.

Following this pretest, the second-year medical students were exposed to a 12-week course for four hours per week in the Physician–Patient Relationship. In this course medical students engaged in bedside interviewing. Discussion of the interviews with faculty followed.

Upon completion of this course by the second-year students, which the first-year students did not take, the test of "clinical judgment" was readministered to both groups. While there was no significant change in scores for the first-year group, the second-year students did demonstrate a positive and significant change in their ability to accept others.

## METHODS FOR IMPLEMENTING UNDERSTANDING

### Reflection of Feeling

Before defining "reflection of feeling" it will be helpful to distinguish between the *content* and *feeling* aspects of what is said. The following example should clarify this difference.

PATIENT:
This hospitalization will mean I'll have to repeat this semester at school. My wife has been getting pretty impatient waiting to get new furniture until I finish college. She'd like to have a car, too. Now I'm thinking of chucking the whole thing and getting a job. At least my wife would stop nagging about how long we have to wait to get some of the things we want.

NURSE:
How long have you been waiting for things?

PATIENT:
Since we've been married. Two years.

The nurse's attention to the factual *content* of the patient's statement was, in effect, a request for more information. It may have
changed the direction of the patient's thinking. A more appropriate
response might have been:

NURSE:
You feel that what your wife wants doesn't jibe with what you want.

Here, the nurse has attempted to catch the essence of the *feeling*
behind the patient's comment. By reflecting this feeling, the patient
may be able to see it in a new light and, in any case, the way is opened
for him to continue considering his problem.

Reflection of feeling may be defined as the statement, in *fresh*
words, of the essential *attitudes* and *feelings* expressed by the patient.[6]
The word *fresh* is emphasized in the definition because the tendency of
beginners is to "reflect content" in the words already used by the
patient. For example:

PATIENT:
I'm really scared about going to surgery tomorrow.

PHYSICIAN:
You're really scared about going to surgery.

The health professional who simply repeats the words of the patient
should not be surprised if the patient discontinues the interview and
asks, "What's wrong with the way I said it?"

The words *attitudes* and *feelings* are emphasized in the definition
of reflection to indicate that the health worker must attempt to be
sensitive to the underlying emotion rather than just the content of
what the patient has said. The interviewer asks him- or herself what
feelings and attitudes the patient is expressing and avoids over-
emphasis on content. He or she must withhold judgment and the offering of a solution.

The above definition of reflection does not mean that feelings are
intrinsically more important than content. Mirroring for patients their
own underlying feelings is therefore not an end in itself, but rather a
means toward helping them see the dimensions of their problems.

These new perceptions enable patients to reorganize their thinking and to seek appropriate solutions.

### Types of Feelings to Be Identified

Feelings are typically classified as positive, negative, or ambivalent. In the course of a series of interviews, and frequently within a single interview, feelings are likely to change from negative to ambivalent to positive.

Early in the interview, the patient is likely to express primarily negative feelings that center on conflicts and hostilities toward others—employer, parents, spouse, hospital personnel. These are reflected by comments such as "You really resented that occupational therapist when she did that!"

It has been our experience that health professionals have little difficulty identifying negative feelings directed at others; they have greater difficulty when such feelings are directed toward the patient or toward the interviewer. When the patient expresses negative self-feelings, portraying him- or herself as "bad" and worthless, the health professional may wish to rise to the patient's defense and, through an attempt at reassurance, point out that these perceptions are exaggerated. It is usually more helpful when the health worker encourages the patient to recognize these negative self-feelings. Then the patient will not have to continue to protest worthlessness and perhaps can begin to move in more positive directions. Similarly, when negative feelings are directed at the interviewer, the health professional may become defensive rather than understanding. For example, when a patient comments on the time spent in the waiting room, it is of little help to be told only that the physician was delayed by an emergency—and no more. Instead, the physician might say, "I'm sorry to be so late. I was delayed by an emergency. I can understand that you're probably annoyed at having to wait so long." In fact, health workers might well anticipate that patients who have been kept waiting will be annoyed and reflect this annoyance at the beginning of the visit, even when the patient does not comment about it.

Another kind of negative feeling frequently expressed toward the health professional is that of dissatisfaction with the progress of treatment. Here too frank recognition of the dissatisfaction rather than defensiveness is more helpful. Comments such as "You seem to feel that these injections I've been giving you aren't doing the job" help the patient see the health professional as an accepting and understanding person. The patient then is more likely to recognize his or her impatience and be more cooperative in the treatment process.

When negative feelings are consistently recognized and reflected, they tend to be followed by more positive feelings. At first these positive expressions are likely to be highly tentative and ambivalent. For example, a patient who has been expressing hostility toward hospital personnel may now say that, although still angry, he or she is also able to see that delays in meeting needs are understandable. When ambivalent feelings are expressed, it is important for the health professional to reflect both attitudes. To continue to recognize only the negative aspects of opposing attitudes will make it more difficult for the patient to discuss developing positive attitudes. Ambivalent feelings may be reflected in statements such as: "Even though you're disgusted by many of the things your occupational therapist does, you feel that, in some ways, the therapist is helping." "You're still dissatisfied with your progress, yet you feel, too, that you may have expected too much."

Frequently the patient will present ambivalent feelings not as a movement away from completely negative attitudes but as a basic problem, especially when a difficult choice has to be made. In these situations the ambivalence is reflected by statements of the following nature: "You'd like to finish your college work, but you're not sure how your wife will feel about it." "You can see that the operation is necessary, yet you're hesitant about going through with it because of the bad experience you had with your last surgery." The health professional should refrain from giving advice and help the patient consider the alternatives clearly. When the patient finally makes a decision, it is more likely to be the correct one—for this particular patient.

Although positive feelings may be expressed at any time in the interview, most of them emerge after negative and ambivalent feelings have been adequately recognized. Positive feelings are reflected in the same manner as other feelings. The patient need not be praised, just as the patient is not criticized for the expression of negative feelings. Conventional praise may, in effect, be belittling, as though a child were being rewarded for being "good." As they move toward more positive attitudes in problem-solving efforts, patients will sense the professional's support through continued understanding responses.

## Difficulties in Reflecting Feelings

### Identifying Feelings
Although the reflection of feelings appears quite simple in principle, in practice it is not easily learned, since it runs counter to our long experience of responding to content. Students of this method are puzzled as to how to identify feelings. In Chapter 10 we shall discuss this problem in relation to some of the common emotional reactions to illness and

treatment. One rule of thumb may be helpful. The interviewer may ask himself as he listens: "What one word describes the patient's feeling when making that statement?" That word or some variant of it may be the clue to use in the reflection. For example a patient may say: "I try my best when I go to physical therapy, but the therapist keeps pushing me to walk even faster." If the interviewer infers that the most accurate word to describe the patient's feeling is "anger," the reflection might be "You're angry because the therapist doesn't see how hard you're trying."

At times a patient's comment may appear ambiguous, and the interviewer may feel uncertain about the accuracy of the inference. In such cases the interviewer may state reflection tentatively and qualify it with, "Is that what you mean?" The qualifying remark not only demonstrates that the interviewer is attempting to understand but also assists the patient to clarify the apparent ambiguity.

When a patient's comment is so unclear that the interviewer has no inkling of what is being communicated, it is best to ask directly for clarification with a statement such as, "I'm not sure I'm following you there. Could you explain a bit more?" Such a response indicates an effort to be understanding, and not a failure to understand. One should never pretend understanding on the basis of ambiguous or minimal information. The patient may become skeptical or suspicious of "mind reading" under these circumstances!

Although every effort should be made to identify feelings accurately, the effect of an inaccurate reflection will not necessarily be negative if the patient perceives the health professional as trying to understand. For example, a patient tells his nurse, in the course of an interview, of the large number of diagnostic laboratory procedures his physician has ordered for him. The nurse makes the inference that the patient is annoyed and states so in her reflection. The patient counters with, "Oh no! Actually, I'm pleased with his thoroughness." The nurse's comment, even though incorrect, encourages a spontaneous reply because the patient has sensed her empathy.

The reader will have noted that the word "empathy" is used persistently in this text. It might be well to distinguish here between "empathy" and the more familiar "sympathy." "Sympathy" usually means the expression of pity or compassion in an attempt to comfort a relative or friend who is in a painful situation. In the professional situation, as empathy is expressed through reflection, the focus is on the emotions of the patient, not the interviewer, although the latter may well feel deep compassion for the patient. The difference between "empathy" and "sympathy" has elsewhere been described as "feeling *with* the patient, rather than *like* the patient."

### Varying the Introductory Phrase

Another common error of the beginner is to preface each reflection with a stereotyped phrase such as, "You feel . . ." The patient will soon sense this response as mechanical rather than understanding. The introductory phrase to a reflection can be varied in many ways:

> "You think . . ."
> "It seems to you . . ."
> "As I understand it, you seem to be saying . . ."
> "You believe . . ."
> "In other words . . ."
> "I gather that . . ."

This list is offered only as suggested variations. The interviewer who has assimilated the principle of reflection can easily extend it. While self-discipline in all their behavior must become second nature to professionals, constriction in phraseology or gestures can create obvious discomfort for both participants in the interview.

### The Use of an Accurate Vocabulary

Many beginning interviewers tend to overuse a few common adjectives such as "angry" or "frustrated" to describe feelings. This limitation misses the broad range of emotions and its many nuances. "Hurt" may often be more accurate than "angry." "Frustrated" is a highly non-specific word and may cover feelings better described as a sense of inadequacy, guilt, loneliness, fear, or confusion.

Further, feelings vary in intensity and in offering a reflection to a patient the interviewer should attempt to capture the degree of the feeling, too. Anger may vary from simple annoyance to real fury. Happiness may range from a placid sense of satisfaction to the heights of ecstasy. Students will readily recognize how helpful an extended and enriched vocabulary can be in practice.

## Acceptance

The concept of acceptance, discussed above, can be communicated in several concrete ways. Although reflection of feeling is the primary method for conveying understanding, it is usefully supplemented by an accepting acknowledgment of what the patient is saying. The health professional responds with, "I understand," "Yes, go on," "I see," "Mm-hm." The same kind of response may also be communicated nonverbally, by no more than a positive nodding of the head, if the patient senses the interviewer's concentrated attention.

The interviewer may sometimes find it useful to repeat a *key phrase* from the patient's statement. For example, a patient concludes with, ". . . and so I was forced to resign from my job." If the interviewer says, "Forced to resign?" the patient usually will elaborate on something he or she has already indicated a willingness to discuss, frequently giving information that might not be forthcoming from direct questions.

Acceptance techniques are particularly useful when the patient is producing material that might arouse feelings of shame or guilt. When the patient perceives that these revelations are readily accepted, the tension that might otherwise be experienced is reduced, and there is more freedom of expression.

As previously emphasized, acceptance is not equated with either agreement or approval. In fact, agreement and approval have more in common with evaluative responses than with understanding. The health professional's function is not to agree or to approve, thereby subtly influencing the patient's decision. The understanding response seeks instead to encourage exploration and, eventually, responsible choice by the patient.

## Interviewer Activity

The importance of attentive listening and the avoidance of excessive or irrelevant verbalization (Chapter 2) have been repeatedly emphasized. It is equally important to emphasize that we do *not* equate these characteristics of good interviewing with passivity. The professional who is listening with concentration, encouraging the patient to speak freely, and making every effort to understand is in reality actively participating every step of the way with the patient. There is the possibility, of course, that the focus on understanding the patient's behavior and verbalization of the problem may at times keep the interviewer silent for longer periods than is comfortable for the patient. The professional must avoid both prolonged silence and oververbalization by appropriate commentary on the patient's communication. Research findings[8,9] suggest that an excessively silent interviewer creates anxiety or resentment. The findings also confirm the point of view just expressed: the successful interviewer achieves a balance between verbalization and silence.

## Reflection and Acceptance of Silence

In Chapter 2 we pointed out that, traditionally, health professionals tend to associate helpfulness with verbal productivity. Consequently when pauses occur in their interviews, they may feel that they are not doing enough for the patient. In addition we have already noted that communication skills brought to the interview tend to be those of social conversation, where pauses cause discomfort and embarrassment. For these reasons, silence in the context of interviews merits special consideration.

Silence, or a pause, can best be understood in the context in which it occurs. For example, in an initial contact with a member of the health professions, a pause is likely to represent a patient's difficulty in getting started. In such cases a brief reflection of this difficulty on the part of the interviewer usually will help the patient begin. In other situations, interviewer silence is appropriate when the patient pauses in an apparent search for words or in an attempt to clarify thoughts or feelings. To interrupt would interfere with the struggle to organize what the patient may be about to disclose. In addition, breaking in might be interpreted by the patient as impatience on the part of the interviewer. It requires as high a degree of sensitivity to know when to remain quiet as it does to make the appropriate remark.

Silence may also indicate embarrassment over discussion of certain topics. Here the health worker might comment, "This is something that's hard for you to talk about." Comments such as these typically encourage the patient to go on talking, since the patient senses the interviewer's recognition and acceptance of unspoken attitudes.

Frequently the patient will express attitudes on a certain subject quite fully and openly and then come to rather an abrupt halt. This pause probably means that the patient has said all that he or she is ready to reveal at the time and is deciding whether to go on. It would be unwise to divert the interview to another topic at this point, since it may lead to the discussion of relatively unproductive material. Rather, the health professional might best remain silent while the patient decides whether to continue. If the pause continues to the point of discomfort for either of the participants, the health worker might attempt to help the patient by commenting, "You're having trouble going on with this, aren't you?"

Silence is also appropriate when the patient appears to be contemplating a reflection of feeling made by the health professional. To interrupt this contemplation might divert the patient from fully assimilating what has been said.

There are times, of course, when interviewer silence may be quite inappropriate. For example, long silences generally are not effective with patients who tend to be distrustful and evasive and serve only to increase distance between interviewer and patient. Further, when a patient demonstrates intense anxiety about his or her complaints, eg,

"I hope it's not my heart, Doctor. My two older brothers died of heart attacks," interviewer silence may be misunderstood by the patient as confirmation of this fear. It would be more useful to comment, "I can see that you're pretty worried about it," thus recognizing the patient's fear and encouraging further discussion.

## Paraphrasing Content

Frequently content and feeling are so interwoven that it would be extremely difficult to disentangle one from the other. Nor is it always necessary to do so. Content is a statement of the circumstances of an individual's life. When these circumstances are so unfavorable that the person needs help in facing or changing them, feeling is inevitably involved.

There may be times when the simple paraphrasing of content, without reference to the feelings involved, may be quite appropriate. For example, the patient's communication may seem confused and jumbled, as in the following interchange:

PATIENT:
You can learn to live with being blind, but you never really get used to it. I know it's not clear, but that's the best way I can express it.

INTERVIEWER:
What I think you are saying is that even though it's possible to manage the routines of living as a blind person, you know that things will never be the way they were. Is that what you mean?

PATIENT:
Yes. That's right. I can manage getting around all right. I'm even retraining for a job. It's the other things that are hard to get used to. No more going to art galleries, no movies or TV, no scenery, and all that.

By paraphrasing the content, the interviewer was able to check the accuracy of his perceptions, knowing that before he can help the patient, he will need to understand clearly the circumstances being described. Having clarified those, he can now go on to deal with the despair this patient is feeling.

On occasion, a patient may feel threatened by a discussion of feelings early in a contact. In such a case it may be useful to concentrate on paraphrasing content.

## Working With Groups

In hospital settings, it has been found increasingly useful for groups of patients to meet with a member of the professional staff to discuss their common concerns. In addition to having their feelings recognized and clarified, patients have the opportunity to perceive that they are not alone and that others have similar problems.

For example, a nurse formed such a group for patients admitted to a public hospital for elective surgery. Patients were available for an average of three or four days prior to their operations. She organized the group to provide its members with an opportunity to discuss their anxieties about impending surgery. The daily sessions were tape recorded, and we reproduce here the serial verbatim statements of one member from each of three sessions:

### FIRST GROUP SESSION

"I don't like the idea of going to surgery but I'm going to go anyhow. I have a lot of confidence in the doctor and I think everything will come out all right."

"The doctors know what they're doing all right. They're interested in you, and I have a lot of confidence in them."

"That's right. The doctors today know a lot more than they did 25 years ago. I wouldn't want any of these old duffers operating on me."

"The doctors told me about my problem."

### SECOND GROUP SESSION

"That's right, and it's not only confidence in the doctor, but confidence in the Good Lord above. I know that between the two of them they're not going to be able to make me look like a Tyrone Power, as I said, but they will make my face a little more presentable."

"Another thing I like about the doctors here is that they tell you about the operation. They tell you the seriousness of it, the exact nature of what they're going to do. They sit down and make a pencil diagram of exactly what is going to happen, which is a very good thing. It gives you some added confidence."

"I know it's going to be a miserable couple of days afterwards, but knowing that the operation will go on all right, I don't mind this so much. I'm not very brave about suffering pain or anything like that."

"Well, I'll tell you one thing. Sometimes I feel pretty good. I don't feel scared. I don't even think much about what's going to happen. But at other times, though, I'm pretty nervous and shook up over this. That's just the way it goes—sometimes I am and sometimes I'm not."

"As near as I can put it, it's like a crap game. There's always a little bit of chance involved in an operation."

"I have some doubts but it doesn't make me real afraid. It makes me a little upset at times, but I'm pretty sure things are going to come out all right, but I do have my doubts at times."

"I wouldn't exactly say I was afraid. But I'm certainly not looking forward to it. And I must admit I get a little scared at times."

"Some people say they're not scared when they go to surgery. Why, they wouldn't be human if they weren't. It's only natural to be scared, and I'll tell you I'm scared."

**THIRD GROUP SESSION**
"I know it has to be done, but it's that waiting around that gets me. If you have a nervous disposition like I do, it can really make you nervous."

"Yes, because I spent the last couple of years in hospitals and having operations, and this is the first time I have ever encountered this conference system. Usually they have a doctor or a bunch of doctors try to tell you what the operation is all about. They sort of try to educate you. They don't give you much of a chance to talk, and they sure don't seem to care about the feelings like you do in here."

"At first, I thought maybe you felt we were all off our rockers, but I can tell by the way you talk to us and treat us that you don't think that. You seem to be interested in us and how we feel about surgery."

"I think we should have these conferences both before and after going into surgery."

"Before we quit, I'd like to say that I'm going to surgery tomorrow, and I think this has helped me a lot. I'm glad that what we have been talking about has been put on tape so that maybe in the future patients can listen to this and get some help. I think especially the nervous type like myself need this a lot."

In this series of consecutive statements, we can observe some major shifts in attitudes. In the first session the patient's comments are limited to his faith in the doctors. By the second session he adds the "Good Lord" to the surgeon's team. In the middle of the second session, he becomes ambivalent: he is not "real afraid," just a "little upset." By the end of the second session, he is openly admitting and accepting his real fear. Further, there is a notable shift in his attitude toward his preparation for surgery. At the close of the first session, he states that "The doctors tell me about my problem." He elaborates in the second session, offering praise for the rational and educational explanations of the surgery; the pencil diagram gives him "added confidence." But in the third session, he withdraws the earlier commendation and instead offers a mild condemnation—"They sort of educate you. They [the doctors] don't give you much of a chance to talk, and they sure don't seem to care about the feelings like you do in here."

We should note that in the earlier discussion of classification of feelings we observed that patients generally move from negative to ambivalent to positive expression. Our patient in the above-quoted group discussion seems to contradict this formulation: first he states his great confidence in the care he is receiving, then he admits to some fear, and finally he is able to express his full anxiety. However, there is no real contradiction. His early statement of confidence in his surgeons is a patent attempt at self-reassurance and denial of his fear. His statements by the third session show growth in his ability to face his anxiety and a new freedom and self-confidence in expressing himself.

The opportunities for initiating such group meetings seem limited only by the ingenuity of professional staff. Many possibilities immediately suggest themselves: providing an opportunity for primiparae to express their anxieties about leaving the hospital and caring for their babies without professionals in constant attendance, giving mothers of chronic asthmatic children a chance to vent their confusion resulting from differing medical views, allowing recent amputees to discuss the readjustments they must make, etc, etc.


## CONGRUENCE OF PROFESSIONAL ATTITUDES AND SKILLS

The above discussion has concerned itself with the principles and methods or skills used in implementing an understanding approach to the patient. This emphasis on "techniques" is incomplete without a complementary consideration of the underlying attitudes of professionals. Physicians and nurses preoccupied with "technique" are not likely to be successful unless these methods are in agreement with their real convictions. "Techniques" sometimes can be mastered almost as rote learning. In the absence of true empathic attitudes, however, skill in the use of words can become a routine exercise that cannot "reach" the patient. On the other hand, health workers who may have sincere and appropriate attitudes may be equally unsuccessful if their attitudes are not implemented by corresponding methods or techniques. Both attitudes and skills must be congruent, neither mere intellectualizations nor lip service to popular theory.

Obviously, most health workers will find themselves at some distance from a fully congruent position. The assimilation of these principles, the development of appropriate professional attitudes, and their integration in operational skills cannot be achieved all at once. In our work with medical and nursing students, we have found that they adopt these attitudes only tentatively and partially at first. As they experience some success, they become more convinced that patients can effectively handle responsibility for their own choices and behavior. If this approach to patients becomes intelligible to practitioners, congruence in method and attitude evolve by gradual confirmation through experience.

## THE USE OF UNDERSTANDING BEYOND
## THE RESPONSE

In discussions of interviewing, skepticism is often expressed that the understanding response—no matter how accepting, no matter how accurately reflective—can, in and of itself, help patients view their problems more realistically and cope with them more effectively. The skepticism is in part justified if the response is viewed in its most limited sense—as one kind of answer to whatever the patient is saying. Questions are often raised, too, regarding the emphasis on feelings. Does this emphasis preclude facing and dealing with problems that in fact do exist, regardless of the feelings about them?

Our meaning has been quite the contrary. We view "understanding" in a broad rather than a limited sense, intended to facilitate change and movement toward problem solving within the patient's capacity to do so. "Understanding" in this sense expands to use related methods (eg, clarification when there are inconsistencies) in accomplishing change and avoiding a static, repetitive fixation on the problem and associated feelings. In succeeding chapters (Interviewing the Family, Counseling), we will discuss the logical extensions of the understanding response which can serve these purposes.

## SUMMARY

The understanding response is defined as one in which the health professional attempts to comprehend the patient's point of view and to communicate that comprehension to the patient. The skills and attitudes required to create an understanding relationship with patients cannot be assumed to result from general professional experience. Although there is some skepticism that these skills can be taught and learned, several research studies indicate that both nursing and medical students do modify their attitudes in a positive direction when exposed to appropriate training.

Reflection of feeling is the primary method for implementing an understanding approach to the patient. This skill is defined as the health professional's statement, in fresh words, of the essential attitudes and feelings (rather than the content) expressed by the patient. In the course of a series of interviews, and frequently within a single interview, feelings are likely to change from negative to ambivalent to positive. Negative feelings tend to be identified readily when they are directed at others. Health workers have greater difficulty when negative feelings are directed at the self or toward the interviewer.

When ambivalent feelings are expressed, it is important to reflect both attitudes. To continue to recognize only the negative aspects of opposing attitudes will make it more difficult for the patient to discuss the developing positive attitudes. To promote the patient's self-understanding, the patient need not be praised when positive attitudes emerge, just as patients are not criticized for expressing negative feelings.

To help in the accurate identification of feelings, the interviewer decides on a word describing an emotion that best captures the essence of the patient's feeling. That word, or some variant of it, may then be used in the reflection. It is also important for the interviewer to avoid using a stereotyped phrase as a preface to each reflection. Similarly, the interviewer should attempt to capture the intensity of the patient's feelings with some degree of accuracy rather than repetitive use of common words like "angry" or "frustrated."

Reflection of feeling in words is usefully supplemented by accepting acknowledgment of what the patient is saying. It is again emphasized that acceptance is not equated with either agreement or approval.

The interviewer is never passive, and always actively trying to understand and encourage the patient's verbalization. However, prolonged silence can create anxiety; therefore the professional must achieve a balance between verbalization and silence. Silence can be useful, however, when an effort is made to understand the meaning of the silence and the context in which it occurs.

Paraphrasing of content may be used when the interviewer wishes to check on his or her perception of the patient's message, or when a patient is threatened by a discussion of feelings.

In a hospital setting it has been found increasingly beneficial for groups of patients to meet with a member of the professional staff to discuss their common concerns.

Finally it was emphasized that, for successful practice of the understanding response, the health professional's attitudes must be congruent with that professional's techniques and skills. "Understanding" is used in a broad sense, rather than the limited sense of an answer to what a patient says. In this context, it is meant to facilitate change and problem solving.

# REFERENCES

1. Adorno TW, Frenkel-Brunswik E, Levinson D, Sanford RN: The Authoritarian Personality. New York, Harper & Row, 1950
2. Ashby JD, Ford DH, Guerney BG Jr, Guerney LF, Snyder WU: Effects on clients of a reflective and a leading type of psychotherapy. Psychol Monogr 71:1, 1957
3. Bernstein L: Teaching counseling skills to medical students. Patient Counseling Health Educ 1:30, 1978
4. Bernstein L, Brophy ML, McCarthy MJ, Roepe RL: Teaching nurse–patient relationships: an experimental study. Nurs Res 3:80, 1954
5. Bernstein L, Headlee R, Jackson B: Changes in "acceptance of others" resulting from a course in the physician-patient relationship. Br J Med Educ 4:65, 1970
6. Brammer LM, Shostrom EL: Therapeutic Counseling, 2nd ed. Englewood Cliffs, Prentice-Hall, 1968
7. Lee H: To Kill a Mockingbird. New York, Popular Library, 1960
8. Lennard HL, Bernstein A: The Anatomy of Psychotherapy: Systems of Communication and Expectation. New York, Columbia Univ Press, 1960
9. Matarazzo JD, Weins AN: Speech behavior as an objective correlate of empathy and outcome in interview and psychotherapy research. Behav Modification 1:453, 1977
10. Shields MR: A project for curriculum improvement. Nurs Res 1:4, 1952

# chapter 8

# Interviewing the Family

In the discussion in Chapter 1 of the family practice specialty, the influence of the family on health and illness was emphasized. Increasingly, this concept leads to working with the whole family together in preventive and treatment programs. We cited a recommendation by Rakel[3] to the family physician that, at an early point in contact with the family, the doctor arrange an interview at which all members are present. This type of "get-acquainted" meeting is meant to serve as the basis for ongoing relationships. It is only one of several possible situations in which it would be important for the physician to meet with the whole family. Other occasions might be times of crises, eg, the onset of a disabling or terminal illness or a death; family situations in which the illness of one member imposes changes on all members, say, in caring for a severely allergic or diabetic child; or perhaps when it is necessary to rearrange the home and individual schedules to accommodate an aged relative. It goes without saying that health professionals other than family physicians will have reason to see whole families together.

In these situations the professional will find that interviewing takes on new dimensions. Specifically, it means that rather than concentrating on understanding one individual, one must be aware of several at once and, in addition, their interactions with one another, as well as with the interviewer.[2] No easy task! However, the principles already discussed, particularly those of the understanding response, remain applicable, even though the presence and participation of several persons instead of only one require a different approach. The interviewer will need to strike a balance between response to each individual and sensitivity to what is in the interest of the family as a whole. This shift in focus to the whole family does not necessarily mean neglect of the individual, since each member will benefit if the family as a whole improves its interrelationships and functioning. There may actually be an advantage to troubled individuals if professionals see them with their families. The interactions may lead more quickly and clearly to diagnostic and treatment formulations.

## RECENT INTEREST IN FAMILY INTERVIEWING IN MEDICINE

It is not an entirely new phenomenon for a doctor or nurse to see two or more family members together. It is a relatively new development, however, that these meetings should be planned rather than occur by chance. Chance encounters between health personnel and patients' families continue to occur, of course. The alert professional can use these to learn a good deal about family interaction, leading, when appropriate, to planned meetings. Observations of behavior then become disciplined rather than casual, so that what is observed can be used constructively in work with the family. Also, when the meeting is held by mutual agreement rather than happening accidentally, its purpose can be stated explicitly and the family can begin to mobilize its resources to deal with its problem.

Education in family dynamics and the behavioral sciences accounts in part for a changing practice that seeks to make positive use of the family's resources in coping with illness and promoting health. As noted above, the practitioner who uses the understanding response has a reliable tool in moving from the individual to the multiple interview.

## SKILLS USED IN FAMILY INTERVIEWING

As with an individual patient, the professional will try to communicate acceptance and empathy from the beginning. At the start of the first interview, the professional makes contact with each member of the family by greeting the individual by name. If they are meeting in the office or in the hospital, privacy and freedom from interruption must be ensured. A meeting in the home is often desirable. The professional might help them begin by a brief statement of the reason for the interview ("We're getting together today to talk about your wife and mother going home, now that she is almost recovered from her operation") and will encourage each member, particularly the silent ones, to express themselves about the matter under discussion ("John, you've been quiet until now. What do you think about your mother coming home?") and see that each has a chance to speak without interruption ("Anne, could we come back to that in a few minutes when John has finished?"). The professional will reflect hostile as well as other feelings, rather than attempt to prevent their expression ("Susan, you sound pretty bitter about all the work you had to do while your mother was sick and feel that John and Anne did not help enough. Do you wonder what will happen when mother gets home, not quite well?"). He or she will be sensitive to alliances and antagonisms within the family and make appropriate comment about them as they affect the problem-solving process ("Mr. T, I've noticed that you and Susan usually agree, but that John and Anne seem not to go along. For instance, you and Susan want Mrs. T to use the downstairs bedroom until she gets stronger, but John and Anne think she can go right back to your room and the rest of you go up and down to take care of her. Either way could work, but are there some other things involved that we haven't talked about?"), and will try to clarify issues by asking relevant questions and pointing out inconsistencies ("John, a little while ago, you said you could go along with this idea of dividing up the work. Now you say you don't think it will work. Did you mean you'd be willing to do your share, but that you see other reasons why it won't work?").

When the circumstances are so threatening (eg, an impending death) that the family members are too frightened to speak openly, the professional will help them by verbalizing the anxieties they have been able to express only nonverbally ("I can see how hard this news has hit each one of you. Now that you know that your mother has cancer, naturally you are afraid she will die soon. Would it help if I answered your questions and explained what to expect?"). The calm use of taboo words, such as "cancer" and "die," will help diminish their terror for the family.

The above vignettes indicate another way in which the physician or other professional can help the family in the interview. It is generally agreed that problems develop when communication among family members is poor or confusing. Frequently each is unaware of or misinterprets the behavior and feelings of the others. By relevant questions and clearly stating observations of their interactions, the professional can clarify and specify areas of disagreement or conflict. This process can lead to resolution and the beginning of cooperative problem solving by family members.

As each interview comes to an end, the professional can summarize the discussion and decisions, indicate still unresolved issues, and, if further interviews are to be held, make specific plans with the family for their next meeting.

## "RULES" FOR FAMILY INTERVIEWING

There are a variety of points of view among family interviewers about "rules" for these family meetings. It is generally agreed, although not universally, that it is inappropriate for preschool-age children to attend the sessions. Some professionals limit attendance only to family members living in the same household. Others include whoever else resides in the home, eg, a maid who is "one of the family." Still other practitioners want those who are important to the functioning of the family (married children, grandparents, etc) to participate, even though they may not live in the same house.

Some family interviewers recommend that, before the first meeting with all members, the health professional meet with one or both parents to prepare them, particularly if strong expressions of hostility are expected. Others feel that, unless all members are present, sessions should not be held at all. The "rules" proliferate as there is increased interest in family interviewing. In general, while some basic agreement is needed between interviewer and family, flexibility may be the most useful "rule." Arrangements can then be tailored to the particular problem and goals for the family. Obviously, once an agreement is reached, professional and family members should be expected to keep to it, except for good and sufficient reason.

Phares[2] notes, in regard to family *therapy,* that there is little research evidence to support one method against another. Yet, he points out, the human need that the workers in this field are attempting to meet is pressing. Research should proceed for obvious reasons, but conscientious professionals need not be too hesitant about beginning work with families if they use a thoughtful approach and avail themselves of opportunities to consult with experienced practitioners and the extensive literature in this field. The same comments apply equally to family *interviewing* in medical practice.

## PROBLEMS IN FAMILY INTERVIEWING

In all interviewing there are potential pitfalls, difficult but not impossible to handle if the professional is "forewarned." In family interviewing, certain problems can often be anticipated.

We have already mentioned the alliances and antagonisms in a family that may become evident as an interview progresses. These can usually be handled by the acceptance and reflection of feelings so often recommended here and by encouraging clarification when, by "taking sides," some members of the family block problem solving. The greater difficulty occurs when, overtly or subtly, one or more members try to win the professional to one side against the other. He or she must avoid rejecting those family members while, obviously, also avoiding actually taking sides. Success is most likely with this kind of family if the professional maintains integrity by continuing to demonstrate acceptance without necessarily agreeing with either side and by verbalizing the conflicts in the family as they become clear.

Another typical problem is the request of one or another family member for individual interviews, often with the intimation that there are matters (family secrets) so sensitive that they cannot be openly discussed. The professional consensus on this issue is that the interviewer should not agree to these individual requests if already committed to meetings with the family as a whole. He or she can avoid rejection of this particular member of the family by giving recognition of the need at times for individual help and offering referral to another professional.

The perennially hostile, somewhat paranoid individual can also create a serious impasse by repetitive disagreement, constant challenges, and expressed doubt of the professional's sincerity. When consistent acceptance of this behavior and the feelings that cause it have no visible effect and when the agreed-upon focus is a more generalized family problem, it seems reasonable for the professional to consider with the family whether continuing under these circumstances is worthwhile. Again, there is the possibility of referral for the disturbed—and disturbing—family member.

The occasional incident of violence in a family interview can be, to understate the matter, extremely disruptive. A family and marriage counselor reported to us the following experience in a first interview with an entire family, the parents and five boys ranging in age from 7 to 15. She had had two prior interviews with the parents alone; the decision to work with the whole family had been mutual. She had been aware from statements of the mother that the father had a bad temper and often used corporal punishment in disciplining the boys. In the interview with the whole family, the 13-year-old, a frail, undersized boy, had been persistently provocative toward the father, whose anger was becoming visible in a flushed face and clenched fists. The counselor was just beginning to point out that the boy was deliberately provoking the father, when the child again made an insulting, sarcastic remark. At this point the father, clearly enraged, jumped from his chair toward the boy, who at the same moment sprang from his chair and dashed out of the room and the building. It was futile to continue with the interview, since everyone became concerned about the boy's safety.

The obvious message in this case is that, while the verbal expression of violent feeling is permissible, acting out is not. Johnny's provocative remarks might have been stopped by a kindly but firm comment such as: "You've already made it clear how you feel, Johnny. If you keep on, trouble may start. Do you want that?" And to the father: "I can see how the hassles you describe begin. Can we talk about another way to handle them?" In other words, in apparent contradiction to the usual goal of self-expression in counseling situations, definite limits must be set on violent, acting-out behavior. The contradiction is more apparent than real, since once disruption occurs it may be impossible to resume constructive work with the family.

Perhaps a word of caution is advisable when family interviewing is being considered. It must be acknowledged that some families are already so disrupted and so unable to relate even minimally to one another that attempts to bring them together may at best be futile and at worst harmful.[2] The interviewer must weigh such factors as extreme resistance to the suggestion of family interviews, overt expressions of strong hostility, long-time absence of contact among family members, and other negative aspects. Under these circumstances, the sick individual may benefit more if the responsible professional interviews individually the relatives who may have some relevant information or some helpful service to offer.

As already noted, family interviewing is a relatively new field. In the absence of a generally accepted methodology for handling often extremely difficult problems, beginning practitioners may find it frustrating not to see tangible results of their efforts. If there is lack of feedback from the family itself, it may be reassuring to remember, as one worker states it: "The methodology for change is developed in the office, but the actual attempt to change usually takes place outside the office in the 'real world' " (p. 547).[1]

## A FAMILY INTERVIEW

Mr. G, 51, is in the hospital recovering from a moderately severe heart attack suffered two weeks ago. The cardiologist believes that Mr. G has recuperated sufficiently so that planning can begin for his return home. Dr. M, his internist, is concerned about the family conditions and wants to ascertain insofar as he can that Mr. G will be able to follow the recommended regimen at home. Dr. M knows Mrs. G and is aware that she is quite tense and has been very apprehensive about Mr. G's condition. Dr. M has also met the three children (Norman, 23, recently married and not living at home; Debby, 17, a high school senior; and Ralph, 14, a high school freshman), but has had only slight contact with them. Dr. M is aware that the family has had financial problems over the years (Mr. and Mrs. G manage a dry cleaning store, part of a city-wide chain) and also that there has been considerable conflict among its members. A cousin of Mrs. G, an employed widow of 50, Mrs. A, has lived with the family for some years.

It has become routine at this hospital for recovering cardiac patients to participate in a discussion group of four to six sessions in the week prior to discharge. Family conferences are also held, sometimes with the physician in charge, sometimes with a nurse or medical social worker, just before the patient leaves the hospital.

Dr. M has arranged through Mr. and Mrs. G to meet with the family a week before Mr. G is to return home. All three children, as well as Norman's wife, Helen, and Mrs. G's cousin, Mrs. A, are present.

The family is already seated around a table in a small conference room when Dr. M arrives about five minutes late.

DR. M:
I'm sorry to be late. I had a telephone call just as I started down the hall, but now I've asked that we not be disturbed for the next . . .

MR. G (interrupting and taking charge):
That's O.K., Doc. I want you to meet my family. You know my wife; my son, Norman, and his wife, Helen; my daughter, Debby, sniffling as usual (Debby, who has been wiping her eyes, turns away angrily), and my son, Ralph. Oh, I almost forgot, my wife's cousin, Mrs. A. She's lived with us for about five years. Now, what's the reason for this family powwow? (Mr. G's tone is sarcastic. Other family members shift about in their chairs uneasily.)

DR. M (speaks in a quiet, pleasant tone):
Remember our talk a few days ago, Mr. G? (Mr. G nods.) I explained then that staying well now will depend on how you take care of yourself once you get home. We've gone over how many hours a day you can be at the store for the next month or so, your exercise program, your diet and medication, how much rest you'll need, but it's just as important, as you know, to keep the tension down as much as possible. And the family (looking around at them) has a lot to do with that, doesn't it?

MR. G:
Sure. You tell 'em, Doc. They don't listen to me. (Everyone seems uncomfortable. No one comments.)

DR. M (smiling):
I'm not here so much to "tell 'em" as to hear what all of you have to say. You know how things are at home better than I, and you know, too, what Mr. G's health problem is. I'd like you to say how you feel about his coming home now, how you think he'll get along, how his health program will affect each of you. Ask questions, if you like.

MRS. G:
Yes, I'm—well—sort of scared. I remember all too well what went on just before he got sick, how mad he used to get about every little thing. What if it happens all over again?

DR. M:
You believe his getting mad had something to do with his getting sick, Mrs. G? (She nods.) Do you all understand what happens in a heart attack? (Several members shake their heads in the negative. The doctor then explains briefly in lay terms.) Do you understand? (Nods from several members of the family.) Mr. G has made a very good recovery, but it does mean that he's somewhat more likely to have another attack than people who have never had one—unless he follows his program carefully and avoids a lot of tension. (General uneasiness in the family.) Does that bother you, make you feel that changes must be made at home?

MR. G:
Yes, you bet. Changes must be made.

DR. M:
Like what, Mr. G?

MR. G:
Well—like Debby not crying over every little thing.

DEBBY (angrily):
I'm not the only one he fights with. It's everyone. But I get the worst of it.

DR. M:
The worst of it?

DEBBY:
I'm supposed to graduate in June—and I've gotten behind in my work because of all the trouble at home. And I don't have a place to work, no

room of my own like that little squirt has (pointing to Ralph). (At this point, several family members speak at once.)

RALPH:
Well, that's not my fault. Norman moved out when he got married, so I've got the room to myself.

MRS. A (angrily to Debby):
You want me to move in with Ralph? You think it's easy for me to be in the same room with you after a hard day's work? (Turning to Dr. M) Believe me, Doctor, I'd move out tomorrow. Except—Celia (Mrs. G) and I—we're close. We grew up together. And she needs me, especially now.

MRS. G (to Mrs. A):
And you don't need me? Where would you go? You can't be alone. (Turning to Dr. M) You see, Doctor, she lost her husband five years ago. Her only child, her daughter, she's married and lives in B_____ (a city 500 miles away) and Connie (Mrs. A) has a good job here. Why should she move out?

MR. G (mimicking Mrs. G):
Why should she move out? Sure, who would you gossip with and play cards with every evening if Connie weren't there? (Turning to Dr. M) You see, Doctor, that's the way we live. Every night, Connie and my wife in the kitchen playing cards, Ralph and I in the living room watching TV, Debby (sarcastically) who has so much homework to do, in the bathroom in front of the mirror, fixing her hair. That's my family. Norman was smart to get married and get out.

NORMAN:
I know you're still mad at me, Pop, about that. You wanted me to stay home and help out after I graduated and got a pretty good job, but— well—Helen and I wanted to live our own lives.

HELEN:
I offered to help in the store to relieve Mom a little on Saturdays, but I made one mistake and he (Mr. G) ordered me out.

MR. G:
One mistake! You gave a long-time customer the wrong clothes! A thing like that could cost us the store! You see how it is, Doctor.

Everyone in this family has complaints. And me, all I'm trying to do is keep my head above water!

DR. M:
Yes. I can see that everyone does seem to have problems, things that bother each of you. I'm wondering—are these the sort of things that Mrs. G says make you so angry, Mr. G?

MR. G:
Yeah. One thing leads to another and, before you know it, it's a big argument.

DR. M:
Uh huh. Mr. G, what you've had to say today makes it sound as though you're pretty dissatisfied with the way nearly everyone behaves.

MR. G:
Yeah. . . . I'll admit I'm no angel either. I've got a temper. (Everyone reacts to this comment with some form of agreement: nods, short laughs, "I'll say," from Debby.)

DR. M (laughs):
Everyone seems to agree. I'd just like to point out, in view of Mr. G's health, maybe there is some way you could get together on making a few changes that perhaps would make things easier for everyone? Just for example—and it's only an example—is there some way Debby could have a few hours of privacy in the evening to do her homework? Because I gather that, if she doesn't, it's not only hard for her, but for everyone. (Several family members now talk at once.)

RALPH:
Debby, you could use my desk in my room.

MRS. A:
I'd keep out of our room for a few hours, if that's what you want, Debby.

HELEN:
You could come over to our apartment to work, Debby. It's not so far away. Norman would walk you home if you're afraid to go alone after dark.

MR. G (laughing):
See, Debby, not everyone's against you.

DR. M:

This is good . . . that you can get together on something that's bothered all of you. I know there are other matters, too. Would it work to talk them over this way, the way we've been doing here? (A few shrugs, some nods of agreement from the family members.)

DEBBY:

Well, maybe it would. It's better than everybody yelling and getting mad.

MRS. G:

Sure it is. Maybe having an outsider with us helps keep our tempers.

DR. M:

I've been thinking along those lines, too, Mrs. G. I can see it's been hard for each of you. There's a person on our staff here at the hospital, a medical social worker, Mrs. Smith, who does just this kind of thing— helps families straighten out day-to-day living problems when someone's been sick and everyone needs to get together to ease things. Would it be O.K. if I talk with her and find out when she could meet with you? (General nods from the family members.) All right, then, I'll do that. And of course I'll keep working with Mr. G on his health and maybe see the rest of you from time to time.

In the above interview, the Gs quickly reveal themselves as a typically dysfunctional family, each member understandably preoccupied with his or her own grievances. They are disturbed by but unable to cope with the life-threatening situation in their midst. Mr. G is clearly frustrated by his patently unsuccessful attempts to control the family situation and his strained relationships with each member. His problem is an almost classic example of the negative effects on health of persistent conflicts in family life.

In view of the serious threat to Mr. G's health, a less understanding, less accepting physician might have been tempted to lecture this family sternly. Instead, Dr. M encourages expression of their somewhat carping complaints and listens to them attentively and respectfully. He keeps the main focus on Mr. G's health, giving the family important factual information that they can understand, but at the same time he helps them engage in a small but cooperative problem-solving experience. He chooses Debby's grievance, her lack of privacy to do her school work, as the most obvious problem of the moment, and it serves his purpose well—to demonstrate how one member's dissatisfaction causes stress for all members.

In a more harmonious, less bickering family, the referral for continued family sessions might not have been necessary. The family might have been expected to use its brief cooperative effort to change a distressing situation for one of its members as a model for dealing with similar troubles. For the Gs, however, while they seem to jump at the chance to come to Debby's aid, one might deduce that their more typical behavior was demonstrated earlier in the interview. Therefore, Dr. M, aware of his responsibility for Mr. G's health, encourages the family in its recognition of its need for outside help. To leave this family to its own devices after this one interview might have amounted to taking a life-threatening risk for Mr. G. In this brief session with a troubled family, Dr. M may have made as important a contribution to their well-being as his medical care of Mr. G.

## SUMMARY

As there is more and more recognition of the importance of the family to health and illness, health professionals are increasingly working with the whole family together. The principles basic to interviewing, especially those related to the understanding response, are applicable in family situations. However, the professional will need to shift the focus from response to the individual to awareness of the needs of the family as a whole. In turn, as family functioning improves, each member benefits. Education in family dynamics and the behavioral sciences has given impetus to using family interviewing to deal with illness and promote health.

The skills used in family interviewing imply communication of acceptance and empathy. The contribution of each member, including expressions of hostility and anger, are encouraged. The professional clarifies family alliances and antagonisms that impede problem solving, gives clear-cut information about the illness and treatment regimen, and, particularly in life-threatening circumstances, helps the family by verbalizing for them their fears and anxieties. The professional also manages to communicate that the family can rely on him or her to "stand by," even in desperate situations. The professional helps keep the family focused on problem solving by summarizing discussions, reviewing decisions, and indicating unresolved issues as each interview ends.

The many different points of view about methodology in family interviewing result in various "rules" for the meetings. There is as yet little research evidence to support one method against another. Therefore flexibility is advisable, provided professional and family establish a basic agreement for working together and keep to it.

A variety of problems can be anticipated in working with families (eg, family members attempting to engage the professional's support for one side or another in family dissension). The interviewer can best handle these potential pitfalls by persistent use of the principles and skills above discussed.

The case example was chosen, not only to demonstrate appropriate skills, but to emphasize the importance of the family to health, illness, and particularly recovery.

## REFERENCES

1. Brockway BS: Behavioral medicine in family practice: a unifying approach for the assessment and treatment of psychosocial problems. J Fam Pract 6:545, 1978
2. Phares EJ: Clinical Psychology: Concepts, Methods, and Profession, rev ed. Homewood, Ill, Dorsey, 1984
3. Rakel RE: Principles of Family Medicine. Philadelphia, Saunders, 1977

# chapter 9

# Counseling

A survey conducted in 1972 by the American Academy of Family Physicians[11] among 2300 of its members revealed that these doctors spent about 20 percent of their office time counseling patients with emotional problems. Since a high proportion of patients present such problems, it is a moot question as to how much more time could be so spent, given the time, training, and inclination. The majority of physicians believed that their medical schools had not prepared them adequately for counseling; many did seek out continuing education courses.

Seven years later (1979), a survey conducted at the National Conference of Family Practice Residents[10] indicated that these residents ranked counseling skills the most relevant subject matter from the behavioral science sequence. Examination of revised curricula indicates that medical schools have increasingly recognized the need for teaching these skills. Further interest is indicated by the publication, beginning in 1978, of the *Journal of Patient Counseling and Health Education*. As Rakel[9] points out, primary care physicians need to be prepared to deal with emotional problems since patients tend to cast them in the counselor role, prepared or not.

## COUNSELING EFFECTIVENESS IN A MEDICAL SETTING

Follette and Cummings,[3] in their study conducted at the Kaiser Foundation Health Plan in the Northern California Region, have clearly demonstrated the effectiveness of counseling in a medical setting. Three groups of counseling patients and a matched control group in similar emotional distress but not seen in counseling were studied for a six-year period. The three counseling groups were seen as follows: 80 patients for one interview only; 41 patients in short-term counseling with a mean of 6.2 interviews; and 31 long-term patients with a mean of 33.9 interviews. During the first year of the study, before counseling was started, these three groups of patients and the patients in the control group (no counseling) had been found to use the inpatient and outpatient medical facilities more frequently than the average. Use of medical facilities was studied for five additional years following the beginning of counseling. There were significant decreases in the use of these medical facilities by all patients in the three counseling groups, while the rate for the control group remained relatively fixed during the total six-year-period. The most significant declines took place during the second year after the first interview. Further, it was found in the five years of study that the one-interview-only and the short-term-therapy groups required no further interviews to continue a reduced use of medical facilities. The long-term counseling group showed no decline in the use of outpatient facilities; the counseling interviews tended to replace medical visits. However, when use of inpatient facilities for this group was examined, it was found to have declined to the average for the Health Plan patients. Prior to the study, the use of inpatient facilities was several times that of the average. This decrease in hospitalization rate occurred in the first year and remained relatively constant.

The Follette and Cummings study suggests several important points for medical practice. First, it is obvious that patients who are experiencing emotional distress are higher-than-average users of both inpatient and outpatient facilities. This finding supports our statement (Chapter 10, under Life Stress and Disease) that when patients under stress visit their physicians, they do not complain of difficult or intolerable life circumstances but of physical symptoms which they, as well as professionals, view as acceptable bases for seeking care. These are the patients likely to be dismissed because no organic basis for the complaints is found. Yet, because the discomfort continues, the result is increased return visits or seeking help elsewhere.

Equally important are the findings that more than half the patients require only a single interview to relieve their distress and that another 25 percent found relief in two to eight sessions. Even if in other situations more sessions were indicated, how much more humane as well as economical for health professionals to arrange for counseling for these patients sooner rather than later! The time required for counseling is unlikely to be more than that taken up by repeated medical visits. The few patients who require long-term counseling could be referred to more appropriate sources.

## RELEVANT COUNSELING SKILLS

As previously noted, it is not recommended that physicians or other health professionals try to be psychotherapists. Rather, counseling skills are viewed as implementing appropriate medical care when problems in personal, familial, or social life either cause physical symptoms or interfere with the treatment of these symptoms. For many patients, the use of the skills discussed in Chapter 7, The Understanding Response, will serve to relieve the immediate stress enough to help the patient move ahead. For example, when the hostility of the shoe salesman who had an ear problem (Chapter 4) was not countered by reciprocal hostility from the doctor but instead was handled with acceptance and understanding, this patient recognized that his anger was based on fear and previous frustrations with medical care. He then became a cooperative patient. Similarly, Mrs. Carson (Chapter 5) was able to decide for herself that avoiding the recommended surgery was "silly" after the nurse provided an opportunity to discuss her confused feelings about her cerebral-palsied son.

In the above situations, the use of an understanding approach helped each patient take a step, however small, toward problem solving. On the other hand, there are some patients who appear to be in a blind alley, who, although clearly troubled and sometimes handicapped by their problems, seem unable or unwilling to change. They tend to deny or blame their problems on others or unfavorable, unchangeable circumstances. Obviously, to continue indefinitely in this kind of impasse is futile. To help such patients, additional skills requiring adaptations and extensions of the understanding response will be needed. These skills might be classified and presented in a variety of ways. In keeping with the general theme of this text, we will discuss them in the following terms: clarification; interpretation; dealing with discrepancies; examining, with the patient, use of the counseling situation; and limits on time. These skills tend to be more successful when a positive relationship has already been established.

Primary care physicians report that, of the problems they see that require counseling, marital discord and difficulties relating to employment are the most frequent. Therefore we will draw on problem situations in these areas for illustrative purposes.

## Clarification

Clarification, by definition the process of making clear, is used when the patient, through confusion, unmanageable stress, or unconscious conflicts, handles a problem in an inconsistent manner or views it in a distorted way. If unconscious conflicts are involved, the patient may even resist change, although suffering real distress. To clarify with the patient the actual issues and dimensions of the problem may be the most important aspect of counseling.

A patient in his late thirties, under an internist's care for a duodenal ulcer, has been complaining repetitively of his wife's lack of appreciation for his efforts to please her. He has also resisted the doctor's suggestion of including his wife in the counseling sessions. He now adds another example:

PATIENT:
I don't understand why she says I don't care for her. I had to work hard and go without things myself to buy that fur coat for her birthday.

Two of the many possible responses might be:

DOCTOR A:
It hurts you not to have her appreciate your gifts.

DOCTOR B:
It hurts you not to have her appreciate your gifts. But, Mr. L, I wonder if you can see some reason for her saying that you don't care for her, although you do buy so many things for her. Do you suppose she means she wants more of your time, your attention?

Dr. A has given an adequate understanding response. However, since the patient's complaint is still another in a continuing series with no indication that he sees himself playing a part in the marital problem, Dr. B goes beyond an understanding answer and offers an alternative idea, a clarification of the wife's atittude. His purpose, of course, is to help the patient move from repetitive complaining to a view of the marital problem that may prove more hopeful. The patient responds, after a few moments of thought:

PATIENT:
Maybe you're right. Just buying things for her doesn't make up for being away so much, I guess. You know . . . the business trips . . . and then the last time I went on that fishing trip, she was pretty mad. Didn't even look at the bracelet I brought home for her. Still . . . I don't know . . . you'd think she could see I need that relaxation . . . you

know, your idea that she should come with me to these sessions . . .
Could we still do that?

This patient may now be past the roadblock of carping, negative criticism of his wife. He is beginning to see her side and is willing to include her in the counseling sessions. The process may now move forward.

Another useful method of clarification is to bring bits of seemingly unrelated material into a unifying theme. Consider the following example:

PATIENT:
I'm trying to do a good job at work, but I have such a hard time with my supervisor. When I do something well, he takes the credit, but if something goes wrong, all hell breaks loose.

COUNSELOR:
Mr. S, I know you feel you get the worst of it with your supervisor. Does this seem to you something like what happened with your father when you were a boy—never able to please him, always being bawled out? And didn't you tell me a week or so ago that you once got so furious with your lieutenant in the army that you hit him? Do all these bosses make you feel sort of helpless, the way you say you felt when you were at odds with your father? Is that what makes you so angry in all these cases? Are they all a lot alike?
(The counselor has been careful to keep his tone as kindly as possible. He waits while the patient considers.)

PATIENT:
Yes, I see what you're driving at. You mean I've got a chip on my shoulder about bossy people, bosses, that it goes way back. Now that you mention it, I made a mess of things the other day with the principal, when he wanted to see me about my son's fighting at school. I took my kid's side, didn't want him taken advantage of the way I was. But the principal was really nice about it, wanted me to talk things over with Joey, so he'd get along better with the other kids. (Short laugh.) Maybe Joey and I have the same trouble. Maybe if my Dad had had a talk with me . . . . Yeah, it's that chip on the shoulder all right.

It should be noted that the suggested clarification (of the patient's problem with authority figures) was the counselor's, not the patient's. The patient had provided the material, but it was the counselor who put it together at an appropriate time. Had the counselor suggested difficulties with authority at the first mention of such behavior, the suggestion might not have been so readily accepted; in fact, it might well have been rejected by this somewhat defensive patient. However, when it *was* suggested, not only had the patient related a number of incidents that supported the generalization, but the rapport between patient and counselor was already well established. It is apparent then that *timing* is also a major consideration in using this method.

It is equally important that clarifications be stated in an *empathic* and not an accusatory manner. As in the examples cited, the counselor needs to be aware of the patient's sensitivities and areas of defensiveness. Clarifications are offered, not forced. Statements in the form of questions permit the patient to accept partially or even reject the counselor's formulation without a sidetracking controversy developing.

As noted previously, when a patient's nonverbal behavior—gestures, posture, tone of voice, facial expression—suggests something that has not been verbalized or contradicts what has been verbalized, the interviewer may call this behavior to the patient's attention. The patient can then draw his or her own conclusions. The patient now has the opportunity to disagree with the interviewer's observation and offer his own clarification. However, an accurate and relevant observation is difficult to deny and often permits previously unexpressed or contradictory feelings to come to the surface and be discussed openly.

## Interpretation

The examples just given in which the counselor helped clarify, in the first case, the patient's problem with his wife, in the second, the patient's difficulty with persons in authority, might also serve as illustrations of *interpretation*—that is, the counselor *interprets* the patient's behavior, encouraging the patient to see his or her own part in the problem. In these situations, the cause-and-effect relationships are fairly obvious and the interpretations quite simple. Often, however, the behavior is more complex, the defenses are more deeply entrenched, and the inconsistencies, resistances, and distortions are less readily recognized or acceptable to the patient. The work of interpretation may require persistence and patience. As noted in relation to *clarification,* timing, awareness of the patient's sensitivities, good rapport, and empathy rather than accusation are important.

Defenses often prove the major block to progress in counseling. In the individual's emotional economy, they sometimes serve a usefully protective purpose. Defense mechanisms also operate, usually unconsciously, as a means of controlling anxiety and maintaining a degree of emotional equilibrium, particularly when under stress. For example, the mechanism of denial is often used to keep unacceptable problem situations from conscious awareness. Similarly, by the use of the mechanism of projection, we tend to place the blame for our difficulties on others to avoid the pain of looking within ourselves. However, defense mechanisms used in this manner are self-defeating in the long run since they preclude realistic appraisal of the problem and require an increasingly strong emotional investment. Temporarily they may protect equilibrium, but at the expense of healthy change. It is in the interest of the patient to bring inconsistencies, distortions, etc, to his or her attention under appropriate conditions through relevant interpretation.

## A Case Example

Mr. Q has been under the care of Dr. N, an internist, for the treatment of hypertension for the past six years.

Mr. and Mrs. Q, both previously widowed, have been married for three years. Mr. Q is 53, Mrs. Q, 51. At the time of the marriage, Mrs. Q left her home in the large city where she had lived most of her life to share Mr. Q's home in a small town about 100 miles away. Mr. Q is a partner in a long-established lumber business. When Mrs. Q, who had found herself with time on her hands during the first year of their marriage, expressed a desire to find some interesting occupation, Mr. Q suggested that she use her skill in growing plants to open a small shop in a new shopping center. He even insisted on financing the venture, although Mrs. Q was willing to use funds of her own. Mrs. Q had undertaken the project enthusiastically and the shop had developed successfully. At this time, two-and-a-half years later, she is considering expanding the shop and taking a partner, a friend of many years.

Mr. Q has been a patient of Dr. N for ten years. A few months after the death of his first wife six years ago, Mr. Q complained of symptoms (dizziness, headaches, general body discomfort) that soon led to a diagnosis of hypertension.

During these six years, Dr. N and Mr. Q have developed a close association. Dr. N has seen Mr. Q about once a month, carefully monitoring his blood pressure and medication. He has also been aware of the changes in Mr. Q's life situation and the effects of his fluctuating emotional state on his health: from the onset of his hypertension at the time of his first wife's death through his lonely and withdrawn period of mourning, followed by a period of almost lethargic acceptance and mild depression, and then a renewal of interest and enthusiasm after meeting and eventually marrying the second Mrs. Q. In working with Mr. Q during these years, Dr. N has become quite familiar with his personal characteristics and behavior patterns. Mr. Q tends to exert strong control over any show of feeling before others; he is conscientious and hardworking in his business obligations; he almost never initiates social contacts, even with close relatives or longstanding friends; and he tends to be compliant and eager to please. Dr. N has deduced that Mr. Q, although competent and apparently successful, is very fearful of rebuff or rejection, highly sensitive and defensive. While he controls outward show of feeling, his blood pressure often reveals his inner state of frustration and anger. Consequently, at such times as seem appropriate, Dr. N, who has been consistently accepting and understanding, encourages Mr. Q to express his feelings by sometimes verbalizing for him the misery and frustration the doctor senses his patient is experiencing. For example, the following interchange took place about seven months after the death of the first Mrs. Q.

DR. N:
Your pressure is a little elevated again, Joe. It's not serious, but I'm going to give you a new prescription that I think will help. Tell me how you're managing the rest of your program—you know, the diet, daily walk, rest, avoiding strain.

MR. Q (immediately defensive, irritable):
I'm doing the best I can. It isn't easy. I'm not used to cooking for myself—and that housekeeper just didn't work out. (Then, recovering himself and assuming a deliberately polite tone.) I'm managing, Doctor, and I do try to follow your directions.

DR. N (nodding):
I know you do. Look, Joe, we've known each other a long time and I can see just how hard it's been. It's all right with me if you let loose and say so. I think you keep things bottled up. You know, it would be better for you if you got it off your chest.

MR. Q (interrupting, now somewhat angry):
How? Who cares? Everyone gives me sympathy . . . (in a mimicking voice) "So sorry, Joe," but no one understands, no one cares.

DR. N:
So that you feel pretty alone? (Mr. Q nods.) But specifically, Joe, who do you mean?

For the first time for him, Mr. Q launches into an angry tirade against his son and daughter-in-law and friends of long standing, a couple whom Mr. Q and his late wife used to see often. The essence of his anger is that these people tend now to exclude him from their social activities. Dr. N is aware that Mr. Q's defensive, withdrawn behavior may cause the very reaction he fears, but does not make this interpretation at this time. Instead, in subsequent interviews, Dr. N consistently encourages Mr. Q's expression of his distress and resentment, inquiring about specifics in the incidents reported and eventually clarifying with Mr. Q his habitual anticipation of rebuff, which leads to such unsatisfactory relations with family and friends. Mr. Q begins to view his own behavior with some humor, at one point describing it as his "cut-my-nose-to-spite-my-face act." His blood pressure stabilizes (with occasional variation) at a satisfactory level and he speaks increasingly of activities that indicate less isolation.

About three months before his second marriage, however, Mr. Q's pressure shows a somewhat alarming rise and his behavior is again tense. Discussion then elicits that Mr. Q has met an attractive widow through relatives in the nearby city, would like to propose to her, but is hesitating, again characteristically fearful of rejection. When Dr. N inquires about specific evidence, however, Mr. Q indicates that she is more than likely to accept him. Dr. N then suggests that some other factors may be causing him to hesitate. Soon Mr. Q responds with a bitter tirade against his first wife, the first indication Dr. N has had of these negative feelings. Mr. Q speaks of his endless "catering" to her "whims," his fear that "trouble" would result if he did not constantly give in to her demands. Mr. Q ends by wondering whether "all women are the same." Dr. N recognizes Mr. Q's ambivalence: on the one hand, he wants the security of marriage; on the other, he is afraid of a repetition of the problems in his first marriage. Through discussions of these former problems, Mr. Q again arrives at a recognition that his dread of rejection often leads him to agreement and "catering" contrary to his real feelings. Dr. N suggests he consider alternatives such as open discussion or frank expression of his point of view. Dr. N further indicates that such expression need not be hostile, but can offer the opportunity for a fruitful exchange.

Subsequently, Mr. Q's hypertension remains under good control and evidently his second marriage is proving happy. However, at the time that Mrs. Q begins to consider expansion of her shop. Mr. Q again has an elevated blood pressure and once more indicates obvious distress. Dr. N soon raises the relevant issue:


DR. N:
Something is changing at home, isn't it?

MR. Q (quite sadly):
I guess it's the same thing all over again, Doctor. I really was afraid of
her starting that shop, but, still, I did everything to help her. Now she
wants to expand it, bring that friend of hers here to help her. It'll take
all her time and where will I be? Out in the cold! (As Dr. N starts to
speak.) Oh, I know what you are going to ask. Why did I encourage her
to begin with? I wish I knew, Doctor, I wish I knew.

DR. N:
Perhaps you were more afraid of what might happen if you didn't? (Mr.
Q nods.) Joe, let's see if we can figure this out, what you are really
afraid of. You know yourself how this fear of yours leads to this sort of
trouble for you. Your pressure goes up, everything seems wrong . . .

MR. Q (quite despondently):
Yes . . . and every time it comes down to the same old thing . . . I can't
say "no," I guess. When you get right down to it, I don't know why,
what I'm afraid of.

DR. N:
I'm not sure either, Joe, but I've had a hunch all along that some time,
some place, when you did say "no" something pretty bad happened and
you fear . . .

MR. Q (quite agitated):
And I'm afraid it will happen again. Yes, I've never wanted to talk
about it. . . . You can see how it upsets me.

His hands are shaking and his voice quavers. He tells then,
haltingly, of a time in his first marriage when his wife left him, taking
their infant son, and returned to her parents. The precipitating event
had been his refusal to buy a home on which she had set her heart, but
there had been prior disagreements of a like nature. He recalled his
rage at what she had done, the painful embarrassment she had caused
him at a time when he was struggling to get a foothold in the business
and social community. Eventually a reconciliation had taken place,
but he had never again risked a serious disagreement with her. As he
talks, he recalls an even earlier episode in his life, when his mother left
the family (he was about 10) after a bitter quarrel with his father. She
eventually returned, but he vividly remembers the misery of her
absence.
    Dr. N uses these recollections to make the obvious but clear in-
terpretation: that Mr. Q's fear is of desertion even more than of rejec-

tion, that his agreement in many situations, in contradiction to his real feelings, is based on this fear, but that often, in spite of his agreement, his personal relationships become conflicted and unhappy. Dr. N further suggests that, inasmuch as his health as well as his marriage is at stake, it might be helpful to have several sessions with Mrs. Q present. Subsequently, these take place; Mrs. Q, when she understands Mr. Q's emotional and health reactions better, proves quite cooperative. In a few months, Mr. Q's blood pressure stabilizes again and he reports less tension.

This case, reported in some detail (although actually only a summary of the most relevant interactions between Dr. N and Mr. Q), suggested itself as a clear and productive use of interpretation. Further, this case illustrates several other theses of this text. The physician indicates a high degree of awareness of the implications for his patient's health of his life circumstances and emotional reactions. The value of an ongoing, trusting relationship between doctor and patient and the relevance to health care of counseling as part of the treatment program are demonstrated. It goes without saying that Dr. N well understands his continuing role with a patient whose particular illness requires this kind of persistent, understanding care.

## Dealing with Discrepancies

Observing the discrepancies between what the patient verbalizes and the actual facts of the situation is relatively easy. Dealing with them is not. An obese patient, who is also hypertensive, states to her doctor that she knows how important it is to follow the recommended diet and that she does so. Yet her weight, taken just before her interview, registers an increase of five pounds since her last visit a month ago. A quite attractive teenager, seeing a school counselor because her grades have plummeted, says that all her problems are related to her ugliness. A young factory worker, who mentions his foreman frequently with comments that he "gets along fine" with him, scowls as he makes these statements. A college student, whose grades have been average and below, argues with his advisor that he should go ahead with applications to medical schools. He knows the requirements for admission, but insists he will work harder and do better once he is a medical student.

Each of these individuals is clearly using denial in handling the situation. As noted earlier in this chapter (see discussion under Interpretation), denial may for a time help maintain emotional equilibrium, but, in the long run, interferes with realistic change and is therefore ultimately destructive.

In dealing with this contradictory and self-destructive behavior, the counselor can point out the observed discrepancy and encourage the patient to explore the inconsistencies. This further exploration may help both the counselor and patient understand what it is that the patient is denying. The obese, hypertensive woman may have a life situation that makes food a source of comfort or perhaps her one pleasure. The teenager who insists that she is ugly may be alienating schoolmates and friends by "ugly" behavior. It may be easier for her to blame her "ugliness" for her isolation, rather than her behavior. She is not responsible for her looks; she is for the way she acts. The factory worker can have so much displaced fear of his foreman that he cannot bring himself to speak negatively of him, even in an accepting situation with his doctor. His facial expressions talk for him. The would-be aspirant for medical school, aware that he has disappointed his parents by his poor college record, longs for a redeeming—and impossible—miracle.

Since the counselor will be pointing out material that the patient has been avoiding, focusing on discrepancies should be used only when a good relationship has been established. The patient is more likely to deal with the discrepancy if it is presented in a tentative fashion, such as, "Could it be that . . . " or "You seem to be suggesting . . . " Certainly, the counselor's comments should never be accusatory. Rather, they should invite the patient to explore previously avoided material.

With some patients, humor can be an excellent tool. A laugh enjoyed together can lessen the tension and help the patient see that it is not a life-and-death matter to maintain the denial. The doctor might say to the obese, hypertensive patient with mock puzzlement, "You say you have followed the diet. Do you suppose there's something wrong with my scale?" Again, as with other tools, the counselor must know the patient, what the patient can handle or, on the other hand, what will be disturbing or offensive.

## Examining Together the Patient's Use of the Counseling Situation

In most continuing interactions between professional and patient, there are periods when the counseling sessions become unproductive. Interviews during these periods may be characterized by frequent changing of the subject under discussion, talking of seemingly trivial, unrelated matters, long silences, direct or indirect expressions of negative feelings toward the counselor, and arriving late or missing appointments. When such roadblocks occur, it is futile to pursue the usual efforts to help the patient work on the problem. Rather, if in the best, disinterested judgment of the professional it is in the patient's interest to continue the counseling, the professional can initiate an examination with the patient of the reasons for the disruption of the counseling relationship.

A frequent cause of this disruption, usually temporary, is somewhat as follows: The patient has discussed a highly sensitive personal matter and has agreed that it would be fruitful to continue the discussion during the next visit. However, the patient is late for the next appointment or fails to keep it. In either case, the counselor, in the absence of other evidence, may infer that the patient has been embarrassed by the earlier discussion or is fearful of where further elaboration might lead. These inferences become the basis for the counselor's comment about the lateness or absence. The same inferences might apply even if the patient had kept the appointment but changed the subject whenever the interviewer attempted to reopen the topic of the previous interview. The counselor can then bring this resistance to the patient's attention. The least helpful approach is to ignore the fact that lateness, missing appointments, or changing the subject is indeed resistance. The degree of the resistance is often a measure of the patient's pain, and if it can be lowered or given up, the pain may also be reduced.

At times, the patient may express resentment toward the professional quite directly. For example, a patient who has talked about a difficult personal problem may suddenly retreat and say something like: "I don't know why I'm telling you all this. I really don't like to talk about such personal things." The implication in such statements is that the professional has somehow elicited the information against the patient's will. The counselor can then clarify the real sequence of events and, without counterattack, suggest possible explanations for the patient's feeling.

At other times, anger toward the interviewer may be somewhat indirect. For example, during a session in which a patient appears angry and has spent most of the last two interviews floundering, she says: "After my boss told me that I wouldn't be getting that raise he promised, I decided I'd been a fool to believe him. I guess a lot of men make promises they don't keep. You can't really trust them." The counselor, on the basis of his understanding of this patient and his observation of her change in attitude, might respond: "And maybe right now you're not trusting me. We ought to talk about it and what has made you change."

Not all difficulties in the professional-patient relationship stem from the patient's feelings and attitudes. Sometimes the professional's own behavior may cause negative reactions. Here the principle is the same as when the difficulty is related to patient behavior: make the best inference as to how you may have led the patient to experience difficulty in continuing the interview and acknowledge it. For example: "I can imagine you're upset by my being late today." Or: "Perhaps I seemed shocked at what you've just told me. If so, I can understand your reluctance to go on." In so doing, the professional demonstrates a capacity to handle negative feelings, even those directed toward him or her.

## Limits on Time

We have previously discussed the setting of limits on aspects of a patient's behavior that may be inappropriate or harmful to self or others (Chapter 5). Similarly, an interview should not be prolonged beyond the agreed-upon time. If the regular length of each meeting is, for example, 45 minutes, it is not helpful to allow the patient to go beyond this, even when important new material is brought up near the end of the session. Rather, the interviewer reminds the patient that they can discuss the new topic at their next meeting, since the time is up for today. Obviously, after a session that has been difficult or disturbing for the patient, the counselor need not be rigid in terminating the interview on the exact minute. A little extra time to recover equilibrium will probably have beneficial effects for both patient and counselor.

A patient who is late for a counseling appointment (barring extenuating circumstances) should be seen only for the remainder of the allotted time. The counselor has set aside that time for the patient—no more, no less. The patient is best helped by learning that counseling has predictable and stable limits. The acceptance of limits is an important part of the growth process for all of us.

## FAMILY COUNSELING

Since the primary physician and/or the office nurse will have become acquainted with family members during their continuing care, it should be possible for them to step into the role of family counselor when the occasion arises. Using the skills and attitudes discussed in Chapter 8, Interviewing the Family, and methods discussed in this chapter, the doctor or nurse can usually undertake counseling of families whose problems do not require more specialized help.

To supplement the discussion in Chapter 8, we describe a method that has proved useful in marriage and family counseling. It may be helpful in marital counseling particularly to have the partners enter into an actual contract about areas of contention.[2] For example, the wife may agree to have meals ready on time, while the husband commits himself to reduce his bowling from three nights to once a week. Although trivial on the face of it, such an agreement may have several positive consequences. First, if each lives up to the contract, one partner perceives the other as trying to do something positive to improve the marriage. Also, both partners may sense that if this area of previous bickering can be resolved, other sources of disagreement may be as well.

Rakel[9] reports using a similar method called "bargaining" with entire families. Each family member prepares a list of actions he or she would like to see changed in other family members. By exchanging these lists, "bargaining" begins, each person agreeing to give up one habit or objectionable bit of behavior on the list if another will do likewise. The professional's role is to guide the bargaining and to act as referee. Ultimately most items on each list should be bargained away. The value of this technique lies, not so much in the mechanical nature of the process, but in the discussion it encourages among family members.

## SELECTING CASES FOR COUNSELING

In 1982 a national survey was conducted to determine career satisfaction among the first graduating group of residency-trained family physicians.[7] The vast majority were satisfied both with the work they were doing and their residency training. One source of relative dissatisfaction was the necessity of treating emotional problems that were beyond their training. Earlier, we stated that nonpsychiatric physicians should not attempt to be psychotherapists, and that counseling should be viewed as an adjunct to medical care when life stresses cause physical symptoms or interfere with treatment of illness. Perhaps the physicians in the survey might have experienced greater satisfaction with their counseling efforts if they could have identified those patients most likely to benefit from short-term counseling.

Anstett and Hipskind[1] have developed useful criteria for selecting patients for brief office counseling—4 to 8 sessions of 30 minutes each. Their criteria relate to characteristics of the patient, the problem, the physician, and the patient–physician relationship.

Patient characteristics correlating with successful counseling outcomes are:

1. Demographic: relative youth, attractiveness, verbal ability, intelligence, success in other endeavors.
2. Awareness that the problem is of a psychologic nature.
3. Presence of "signal anxiety" (anxiety focused on changes in self).
4. Personality traits: persevering, dependable, nonimpulsive, trusting.
5. High motivation for change in self.
6. Faith that counseling can be helpful.
7. Awareness of how counseling works.
8. Previous successful counseling experience.
9. A personal resource system supportive of the aims of counseling.
10. Absence of debilitating characterologic components within the personality (eg, severe hypochondriasis or feelings of anger or distrustfulness).
11. Previous meaningful interpersonal relationships.

Problem characteristics correlating with successful counseling outcomes are:

1. The presence of an acute precipitant.
2. A relatively brief duration of the problem.
3. Minimal secondary gain associated with the problem.
4. Minimal somatic components to the problem.

Physician characteristics correlating with successful counseling outcomes are:

1. Ability to empathize with patient and problem.
2. Ability to conceptualize the problem.
3. Belief that the counseling can be helpful.
4. Time to treat the patient's problem.
5. Ability to separate patient's problem from own personal concerns.
6. Ability to establish a working relationship with the patient.

Patient–doctor characteristics correlating with successful counseling outcomes are:

1. Ability of physician and patient to agree on the nature of the problem.
2. Ability of physician and patient to agree on goals of counseling.

3. Ability of physician and patient to agree on the particulars of counseling, ie, the roles to be played by each, the length of counseling, the expense of counseling.

These criteria are intended as useful guidelines. Some of them may be more important than others in predicting success. There is no evidence that a certain number of the criteria must be met.

Using the above guidelines, the professional may choose to refer to other sources those cases that are felt to be beyond his or her preparation.

## REFERRAL

The amount of time health workers devote to counseling will vary according to the nature of their practice and the degree of satisfaction derived from the various aspects of their professional work. Hodges[4] has described a fruitful physician–psychologist collaboration in an office-sharing practice. Others may choose to refer most patients who need counseling to a variety of other sources.

Although it is neither desirable nor possible to refer every patient with emotional problems for psychiatric help, there will be times when referral to a psychiatrist is necessary. The criteria for psychiatric referral have been delineated as follows by Lebensohn[6]:

1. Persistence of incapacitating psychoneurotic symptoms such as phobias, anxieties, obsessions, or hysterical manifestations.
2. Persistence of psychogenic sexual problems.
3. Psychotic symptoms, such as hallucinations or delusions.
4. Sudden change of personality or judgment.
5. Exaggerated swings of mood or motor activity.
6. The development of retardation, depression, or self-destructive thoughts (p. 124).

Physicians frequently overlook the psychiatric aspects of an illness. For example, in one study,[5] 1000 outpatients who presented puzzling diagnostic problems were examined at the New York Mount Sinai Hospital consultation service. In 814 of these cases, a psychiatric diagnosis was made, either as a primary or secondary factor. In only 166 of the 1000 cases was an organic disease without psychologic implications diagnosed. Most striking was the fact that in only seven of the 1000 cases did the referring physician suggest possible emotional factors.

When a decision has been made to refer a patient to a psychiatrist, psychologist, family agency, or other mental health resource, the health worker cannot compromise with honesty. Patients have been told that they are to see nerve specialists, nerve doctors, or neurologists. Lebensohn[7] reports receiving as a referral from a general practitioner a man who complained of body lice. When the physician could find no lice, the patient was referred to a specialist who had a special microscope! Upon arriving at the specialist's office, the patient discovered he was to see a psychiatrist and walked out.

As in any other referral to a specialist, the patient should be told that the purpose is for examination, diagnosis, and possible treatment, without specifying what examination and treatment the specialist will provide. The reasons for the referral should be clarified rather than avoided, and the referring physician should be prepared to discuss the patient's doubts and anxieties about the referral. In the following example the physician has recognized the patient's alarm over a psychiatric referral:

PHYSICIAN:
Your depression hasn't responded to medication, Mr. Jones, and in our talks we haven't been able to come to an understanding of it. It might be helpful for you to see a psychiatrist about this.

PATIENT:
A psychiatrist? I'm not crazy!

PHYSICIAN:
Of course you're not. But the idea of going to a psychiatrist has upset you?

PATIENT:
Well, I suppose he'll use shock therapy.

PHYSICIAN:
He will decide on the treatment after his examination. But you seem to associate all psychiatric treatment with shock. I guess that can be pretty frightening.

PATIENT:
Well, it is. But maybe they only use that on patients who have to be locked up?

PHYSICIAN:

I can well understand your fear. Especially when you've had no experience with psychiatrists.

PATIENT:

Just what I've seen on TV. Sometimes those guys don't seem so bad.

PHYSICIAN:

You're beginning to see that maybe it won't be so frightening. I'll give you Dr. X's and Dr. Y's telephone numbers. You can call one of them after you've had a chance to think it over.

PATIENT:

Thank you, doctor. I guess I'll call one of them.

If and when this patient appears at the psychiatrist's office, he will be better prepared for treatment. His physician accepted his fears and helped the patient understand them. The reader may well contemplate the consequences if the patient had been told he was to see a "nerve specialist" who later turned out to be a psychiatrist. One may also wonder about the outcome had the physician reassured the patient that he would not receive electric shock therapy only to have the psychiatrist recommend such treatment. It is not the function of health workers to predict the care another professional will prescribe. Rather, their responsibility is to explain and help the patient accept the need for specialized treatment.

Although physicians readily make referrals to other medical specialists, the use of community agencies such as family service organizations is much less frequent. Many family service agencies offer the full range of individual, marital, and family counseling services. Such services are not intended only for the indigent; rather these agencies maintain sliding fee schedules, so patients and families with enough money can pay for the help received.

Morgenstern[8] describes an effective referal to a social agency of a family that had been making excessive demands, after it became clear that the family's problems were too severe for the physician to handle alone.

The latest incident involved Mrs. Dawson, who brought Tommy to the office to have a splinter removed. After the splinter had been removed, it was suggested that Tommy stay in the reception room with the receptionist while the physician interviewed Mrs. Dawson in the office.

PHYSICIAN:

Mrs. Dawson, you've been having more than your share of problems with the children for some time now.

MRS. DAWSON:

Yes, I certainly have.

PHYSICIAN:

I think other things are going on at home. I'd like to try to help if I can.

MRS. DAWSON (bursting into tears):

Oh, doctor, you can't imagine how hard it's been. Joe lost his regular job. It's been two months now. He's managed to get a few days each week working on the loading dock, but he hates it. We thought everything would be better when we moved here—it's hard for Joe to make friends. For me too. We don't know *anyone* here. The bills keep coming, and our savings toward the house are going. It just looks so hopeless. Joe doesn't talk to me anymore. He seems to blame me for something. He drinks a lot more than he used to. It's so different between us. I find myself thinking there may be someone else.

PHYSICIAN:

It's affected your marriage, too.

MRS. DAWSON:

Yes! My Joe came up the hard way. He's been on his own since he was sixteen. Something began to happen between us a year, no, almost two years ago now. . . .

Tommy breaks everything he touches. And last week he found some matches and almost set the neighbor's garage on fire. The neighbors were never friendly. Tommy picks on their little girl. His report card was awful this time. I know he's bright. And Julie's getting worse. Now the school wants to see me about both of them. I'm afraid to face them. I feel like such a failure. If only I wasn't so tired all the time. . . .

PHYSICIAN:

It's obvious that things are pretty rough for all of you. Do you think you could get Mr. Dawson to come in with you some day next week?

MRS. DAWSON:

I think so. Why?

PHYSICIAN:

I'm concerned about the children. And you and your husband too. Can you both be here at 6 P.M. on Monday?

Mrs. Dawson agreed. The physician sensed she was feeling emotions of both relief and expectancy. The talk had taken four minutes.

On the following Monday, Mr. Dawson opened the interview.

MR. DAWSON:

Fran didn't say much about why you wanted to see us, except it's about the kids, Doc. They mean more to me than anything.

PHYSICIAN:

Mrs. Dawson told me about your job change. Sounds like it's been pretty rough for you.

MR. DAWSON:

It's been tough all right. I've worked hard my whole damn life. It wasn't right for them to take that new guy. How would you feel if you couldn't bring in more than seventy bucks a week when you're used to more than three times that?

PHYSICIAN:

You feel pretty rotten, and maybe you're wondering what you've done wrong.

MR. DAWSON:

I do. . . . We had almost 2500 bucks saved toward the house, and it's all going down the drain. Everything's wrong lately . . . I guess you know Fran and I aren't getting along.

PHYSICIAN:

Mm-hm.

MR. DAWSON:

I know this has upset the kids. Tommy's getting meaner than a snake. Did Fran tell you about Julie's nightmares?

PHYSICIAN:

No, but it's obvious that the whole family is going through a bad time. Everyone's feelings are all mixed up because of the strain of a recent move and a financial setback that has you all spinning. It's all pretty complicated. It takes time to understand it all. At this point I have only a slight understanding. The big question is, do you want some help? The kind of help that might get the whole Dawson family feeling better?

MR. DAWSON:
What kind of help?

PHYSICIAN:
I'm talking about your seeing some people at an agency that specializes in giving the kind of help your family needs. I'm talking about family counseling—where you'll have the opportunity to talk over your feelings and problems so you can understand them better, and so you can both understand how you affect the kids and how they affect you. But the big thing is that when the two of you are getting along better, the children should start doing better too.

MR. DAWSON:
If Frances is for it, O.K. Anything is better than how we've been living.

An effective referral followed.

## SUMMARY

There is substantial evidence that counseling skills are increasingly considered of first importance by family and other primary-care physicians. These health professionals spend about 20 percent of their time in counseling. However, since a high proportion of patients present problems for which counseling would seem appropriate, it is a moot question as to how much more time could be so spent.

Although it is generally recognized that emotional factors play an important part in illness, these factors are often overlooked in medical diagnosis. Patients may therefore be dismissed if no organic basis for complaints is found. Since these patients still suffer from their symptoms, however, they tend to make additional visits or seek out new physicians, using a disproportionate amount of medical time and services. When appropriate counseling is offered, their use of these services decreases markedly.

For many patients the use of the understanding approach, described in Chapter 7, will provide the necessary service. For other patients, however, additional skills—adaptations and extensions of the understanding response—will be required. These skills are here classified as: clarification, interpretation, and dealing with discrepancies, appropriate in situations where inconsistencies, resistances, and distortions by the patient interfere with problem solving. Essentially the objective of these skills is to help the patient see his or her own part in the problem, thus becoming better able to cope with it. These methods are most successful: (1) if the rapport between professional and patient is well established, (2) when used in an empathic rather than accusatory manner, and (3) when the counselor, aware of the patient's sensitivities and defenses, applies them at an appropriate time.

A further skill helpful in counseling situations that continue over a period of time is used when interviews become unproductive. The patient is not ready to terminate counseling, but the resistances that arise for any of a number of reasons block progress. The professional can then bring to the patient's attention the use he or she is making of the counseling situation. It may be necessary to focus on the resistance itself.

An interview session should not be prolonged beyond the agreed-upon time. However, after a session which has been disturbing to the patient, time to recover equilibrium should be allowed. When late for a counseling session, the patient (barring extenuating circumstances) should be seen only for the remainder of the allotted time. The patient will learn that counseling has stable and predictable limits.

Even skilled counselors will at times need to refer certain patients to specialists, psychiatrists, or community agencies. Criteria for such referrals and illustrative case examples are given. Referrals tend to be most successful when the primary-care physician takes time to clarify the reasons for the referral and helps the patient make the transition to the specialist.

## REFERENCES

1. Anstett R, Hipskind M: Selecting patients for brief office counseling. J Fam Pract 13:186, 1981
2. Bissonette R, MacKenzie JA: Premarital and marital counseling: realistic intervention strategies. In Taylor RB (ed): Family Medicine: Principles and Practice, 2nd ed. New York, Springer-Verlag, 1983
3. Follette WT, Cummings NA: Psychiatric services and medical utilization in a prepaid health plan setting. Med Care 5:25, 1967
4. Hodges A: Psychosocial Counseling in General Medical Practice. Lexington, Mass, DC Heath & Co, 1977
5. Kaufman MR, Bernstein S: A psychiatric evaluation of the problem patient. JAMA 163:108, 1957

6. Lebensohn ZM: Psychiatric referrals: handle with care! Med Econom 48:215, 1971
7. McCraine EW, Hornsby JL, Calvert JC: Practice and career satisfaction among residency trained family physicians: a national survey. J Fam Pract 14:1107, 1982
8. Morgenstern JA: The practitioner and his community. Feelings and their medical significance. Ross Laboratories pp 1–4, 1972
9. Rakel RE: Principles of Family Medicine. Philadelphia, Saunders, 1977
10. Shienwold A, Asken M, Cincotta J: Family practice residents' perceptions of behavioral science training, relevance, and needs. J Fam Pract 8:97, 1979
11. Stanford BJ: Counseling: a prime area for family doctors. Am Fam Physician 5:183, 1972

# chapter 10

# Emotions in Illness
# and Treatment

The significance of feelings in illness and treatment has already been emphasized in discussions of the professional–patient relationship and interviewing methods. Increasingly, the evidence from research and medical observation demonstrates that emotion can be a potent force in causing illness, complicating and/or prolonging it, and reducing the effectiveness of even the most carefully planned treatment. One of the axioms of this text is that responsible care of patients must recognize, understand, and deal appropriately with emotional reactions if optimal benefits are to be obtained.

In this chapter we present a closer examination of the relationship of stress to illness and of those emotional reactions most often encountered in illness. Through use of examples, approaches are suggested that may minimize these untoward effects. Reference will be made to innovations in medical care such as renal dialysis and cardiac surgery, because the very nature of these dramatic advances in formerly fatal illnesses may precipitate reactions that can negate whatever gains the patient might otherwise achieve.

## LIFE STRESS AND DISEASE

### Functional Illness

The widespread popularization of principles of psychosomatic medicine have increased the general awareness that physical symptoms can be caused by emotion. We are all familiar with the tension headache after

a bitter quarrel, the student's nausea and vomiting before an important examination, the pounding of the heart when bad news is heard.
Usually these symptoms disappear soon after the immediate stress
terminates. However, what if the stress is not a single disturbing event
but a life of sequential misery related to continuous family tensions,
frustrations on the job, financial worries, and the like? Under such
circumstances patients are hardly likely to report to the physician that
they cannot tolerate their life circumstances. Rather, they can be expected to appear at the physician's office complaining of vomiting,
headaches, or whatever the symptom. All too frequently such patients
are examined and dismissed because there is no physical basis for their
complaints, which seem temporary or imaginary. Yet "emotional"
vomiting is just as distressing as vomiting caused by an obstruction of
the pylorus; tension headaches are just as painful as those caused by a
brain tumor. Perhaps we need to be reminded that "disease" originally
meant lack of ease. Branch[8] has stated that:

> Medicine has certainly done a spectacular job of coping with
> the noxious elements outside the organism and correcting dif-
> ficulties once they have occurred inside the organism, but the
> present-day killers are found in the way we live and the psy-
> chological and social factors which impinge on our illnesses.
> These are the elements which make the difference between
> suffering and mere pain and which determine the degree to
> which the individual is incapacitated by the illness or injury.
> The degree of incapacity is largely independent of the actual
> amount of pathology present (p. 33).

Many health workers are aware that their training has not
equipped them to treat functional ills with the same degree of competence with which they deal with physical ailments. One study cites 51
percent of physicians as noting deficiencies in their social-psychologic
skills. Awareness of this deficiency is dramatically increased over
time. Forty-three percent of those graduating from medical schools
prior to 1929 and 81 percent of those graduating after 1945 cite such
deficiencies in training.[39]

Health professionals do not need to become psychotherapists to
recognize that taking time to listen and to understand is an important
element in treatment. Bennet[5] has stated that the essentials of improvement and cure for patients with functional illness lie largely in
the relationship between health professional and patient. With the
development of skill in handling these complaints, the professional
will enlarge the scope of healing and benefit a high proportion of pa-

tients—those with purely functional complaints and the many who experience a functional overlay along with their somatic illness.

## Stress Factors in Physiologic Illness

An ingenious series of studies by Holmes and his associates at the University of Washington School of Medicine, reported in summary by Holmes and Masuda,[28] demonstrate quite clearly that clusters of life events are associated with the onset of illness—illness for which there *is* a physiologic basis. In studying thousands of tuberculosis patients, the authors found that these patients suffered a variety of life crises shortly before becoming ill. The investigators then developed a list of 43 life events reported by their patients as requiring varying degrees of readjustment in their lives. It was not unexpected that disease would follow life events of a negative nature—divorce, death of a spouse or close relative, loss of job, etc. What proved to be a surprising and relatively new concept was that ordinary or even desirable changes—vacation, outstanding personal achievement, etc—can also predispose the organism to illness.

Holmes and his colleagues did not conclude that any particular life event triggered a particular disease. The important finding was that the sum of life events, each of which required a degree of coping, caused stress and the stress, illness. They then worked out a method of numerical scoring, ranging from death of a spouse (the most stressful) at 100 points, to marriage (50 points), to outstanding personal achievement (28 points), down to minor violations of the law (11 points). This scale, known as the Social Readjustment Rating Scale, has been found to be reliable and valid in predicting disease. For example, Holmes and Masuda[29] have demonstrated that 85 percent of medical students with high life-change scores had major health problems during the first two years of medical school, in contrast to 33 percent of students with low life-change scores. Life-change events are predictive not only of the onset of illness, but also the course of recovery. For example, a correlation between high levels of life change and poor physical recovery has been found in myocardial infarction cases.[20] In another study of heart attack patients, there was an association between premorbid life-change scores and higher depression and anxiety scores during recovery.[54]

Holmes and Masuda[28] summarize their findings as follows:

> The search showed, then, that human beings do indeed get sick when they have to cope with many of the events of normal

life. When they struggle with overwhelming life crises, they tend to get more serious diseases. The explanation, we suspect, is that the activity of coping can lower resistance to disease, particularly when one's coping techniques are faulty, when they lack relevance to the type of problems to be solved. This approach to illness is a lesson in human finitude. It reminds us that we have only so much energy, no more. If it takes too much effort to cope with the environment, we have less to spare for preventing disease. When life is too hectic and when coping attempts fail, illness is the unhappy result (p. 106).

The demonstrated relationship between life events that strain coping capacities and disease offers the health professional a new avenue to preventive care. At the time of the first office visit, patients could readily complete the rating scale in the waiting room in less than 15 minutes. The health professional can use this information to help high-risk patients avoid all but the most necessary life changes. Health workers who maintain a good relationship with patients will know about the changes facing those under their care. They will be in a position to help with appropriate coping procedures, thereby preserving their patients' energy for preventing disease. For example, investigators at the University of Washington[53] report the case of a 30-year-old man who consulted his family physician complaining of depression and dissatisfaction with his job. At the time of the consultation, the patient, who had been married for two years, reported the birth of a congenitally defective child one month earlier. Six months before the child's birth, he had had a promotion to a position of increased responsibility in the firm where he had been employed for the past five years. Now he was thinking of changing jobs. Examination revealed hypertension in addition to clinical depression. He was started on tricyclic antidepressants and antihypertensive medication. The patient was also asked to fill out the Social Readjustment Rating Scale, which indicated an already dangerously high score. When it was explained that the proposed change in jobs would place him at even increased risk, he decided instead to request a one month's leave of absence to help his wife care for their sick baby. In a later follow-up visit to his doctor, he reported satisfaction in returning to his job. It was possible to reduce the amount of antidepressants and maintain him successfully on the hypertensive medication.

More recently, there has been evidence that attention to significant life changes may be useful in the management of chronic disease. Petrich and Holmes[44] report studies in which cardiac patients who had an opportunity to discuss life changes in brief group therapy sessions returned to work significantly earlier than a control group. They also had significantly lower reinfarction rates than controls.

## EMOTIONAL REACTIONS TO ILLNESS AND TREATMENT

Because the subject matter of emotions is so complex, the use of a conceptual framework is helpful in organizing material that can often seem diffuse and confusing. For our purposes the classification by Senescu[50] has proved applicable and is adapted here. It should be emphasized that all conceptualizations and classifications are inevitably simplifications for the sake of clarity. In practice, feelings will often present themselves in ambiguous, sometimes disguised form. They are nevertheless present as an important factor, and the knowledgeable professional will give careful consideration to their effects on patients' well-being.

In our adaptation of Senescu's classification, we use three groupings of emotional reaction: (1) those that are most likely to manifest themselves as a direct result of the illness or treatment—fear, feelings of damage, and frustration caused by loss of habitual gratification and pleasure; (2) those that the patient brings to the illness from his or her idiosyncratic personality patterns and life-style—an individual way of coping with anger, dependency, and guilt; (3) more serious manifestations—depression and loss of self-esteem, which may emerge particularly if the above-mentioned reactions are not recognized or do not respond favorably to the professional's intervention.

## Emotional Reactions Directly Related to Illness or Treatment

### *Fear and Anxiety*
Fear can be defined as anticipatory dread of pain, danger, or disfigurement. Anxiety usually is at a high level. Fear may be expressed directly or indirectly by repeatedly asking the same questions, demanding attention, or making pleas for reassurance. Fear may also demonstrate itself in physiologic distress: pallor, restlessness, perspiring, muscular tension, stomach upsets, diarrhea or constipation, headaches, etc.

Intense anxiety and fear sap the patient's strength and consume energy that could be used more constructively in combating illness or contributing to recuperation. For example, Klopfer[33] studied the personality differences between patients with fast-growing cancers and those with slow-developing ones by using the Rorschach inkblot test. Patients who demonstrated high ego-defensiveness, typically fearful and anxious persons, tended to have fast-growing cancers. He concluded that the overinvestment of vital energy in ego defenses deprived patients of the resources and energy to fight the onslaught of cancer. Verwoerdt[56] points out that slowly developing illnesses permit greater time for both psychologic and physiologic adaptation, whereas rapidly developing conditions may have an overwhelming effect.

Fear and anxiety may also strain the controls and defenses that are the "glue" of personality. If these controls are disrupted and the patient "goes to pieces," then referral or precautions against even greater danger or possible suicide may be necessary. In any event, such disruption can only complicate the patient's existing physical condition.

Because fear is so debilitating, health professionals should attempt to handle it with the patient as soon as it is recognized. Information concerning the patient's physical condition and planned treatment can be provided in whatever detail the patient is able to assimilate. Emotional support that follows can reduce the level of fear. When information and the understanding methods previously discussed do not suffice to abate the fear, then additional steps must be taken. It may be necessary to confront the patient with this exaggerated or uncontrolled fear in realistic, not hostile, terms. The fear probably will be involved with life circumstances and relationships that have been complicated or aggravated by the illness, as the following example illustrates:

A young man is offered a highly desirable position at an excellent salary with a South American corporation. Shortly before he is to leave to accept the position, he suffers a sudden attack of appendicitis. Surgery is successful and recovery should be unremarkable. However, this young man gives evidence of unusual pain, has a turbulent convalescence, and reacts with antagonism, suspicion, and dissatisfaction to those who care for him. Finally, in bewilderment, the nurse says, "You know, you're not that sick any more. Nothing we do seems to help you. Why don't you tell me what's bothering you?" The patient is disarmed, but he hesitates. The nurse waits. He begins then haltingly to explain. He finally got the kind of job he has always wanted, and is now fearful that because of his illness the offer will be withdrawn. He may be considered too sickly to tolerate the rigors of the work in South America. The nurse listens, accepts by nodding. Further discussion clarifies that accurate medical information from his doctor to his employer will establish the fact that usually his health is excellent. The patient realizes that his concern was an exaggeration. He is relieved. Freedom from this fear, however, does not "free" him. He is still anxious, still restless. He is encouraged to go on by: "There is still something bothering you." He continues in an outpouring of contradictory, angry, defensive complaints. He should not have accepted the new position, even though it is what he really wanted. It's his widowed mother. He is the only one who can take care of her. She "goes into a tailspin" every time he considers employment away from home. Well, now she's going to have to learn to get along without him. She'll have to hire a housekeeper or make other arrangements.

His problem is indeed two-edged. The patient is caught between his longing to leave home and prove himself in a challenging position, and his sense of obligation to his mother. His conflict is acknowledged. It is suggested that perhaps his mother's circumstances can be reappraised and alternative arrangements considered, so that if he does decide to leave he can do so with less worry. He is offered the opportunity to explore his problem further with the hospital social worker. He agrees to this referral. His convalescence then proceeds more smoothly. The nurse's sensitivity to the patient's anxiety has uncovered his underlying fear and conflict. His physical recovery has been facilitated and his psychologic problem may now be further clarified.

Fear and anxiety are common reactions, not only to being ill, but also to certain treatment procedures. Iatrogenic anxiety (anxiety inadvertently precipitated by medical attention) is observed frequently. For example, when blood pressures are taken often, the patient may become concerned that something is wrong of which he has not been informed. The mere fact of undergoing the procedure can raise the blood pressure. A physician's concerned look while listening to the patient's heart, frequent and numerous unexplained laboratory tests, and comments made in the patient's presence during teaching rounds can all arouse anxiety in the patient. The attending professionals need to remember that patients are not objects to be manipulated. Explanations given in understandable and understanding terms will reduce the level of fear and anxiety.

The anxiety of patients undergoing the difficult process of renal dialysis is almost predictable. Even before starting dialysis, these patients have undergone severe stress. In addition to dietary restrictions and a general decline in their physical status, they come to know that their illness is not curable. Death seems always imminent, and living as chronically handicapped persons is almost as fear-inspiring.[51]

Beard[4] found that patients who were able to adjust with relative success to dialysis and to the uncertainty of their futures were those who had a close relationship with a health professional with whom they could discuss their fears when stress and discouragement reached high levels. In one program for these patients,[27] the hospital created the position of a nurse clinician. She had taken special training in renal disease, as well as in concepts of interviewing and professional relationships. Her function is to interpret the physician's instructions to the patient and the family, to coordinate rehabilitation efforts, and to handle difficulties in family adjustment. Her availability as tensions inevitably arise offers an important resource for ventilating feelings, as well as access to services for problems related to the illness.

Blacher and Basch[7] report that cardiac patients about to undergo surgery for pacemaker implantation expressed strong fear of any surgery having to do with the heart. Even those patients who had had a successful first operation expressed a fear of dying in a second procedure to replace batteries. Some were even afraid of falling asleep for fear their hearts might stop. In a survey of 800 patients who had undergone cardiac surgery,[24] most patients expressed a wish for more emotional support than they had been given. As a result of this finding, it is suggested that verbal expressions of anxiety and fear be encouraged at all stages in the operative sequence. Dhooper[17] studied the experiences of 40 families with no history of major illness, where the patients, aged 32–60, were hospitalized with a first myocardial infarction. These families reflected the racial composition and the socioeconomic levels of the city in which the study was conducted (Cleveland, Ohio). Data were collected at the time of hospitalization, a month after discharge, and again three months later. It was found that the immediate impact of the illness aroused marked anxiety in members of the family other than the patient. Even after the patient was considered to be "out of danger," but still in the hospital, the anxiety of the spouses in particular remained high. A month after the patient returned home, 90 percent of the spouses were still experiencing some anxiety about their partners' illness. It was during this period that, in almost 25 percent of the cases, another family member became physically ill. These illnesses were attributed to the emotional strain of the crisis. Three months after discharge, most families had returned to "normal," although most spouses reported that, knowing the patient had permanent heart damage, they continued to feel some anxiety. Although the hospitals participating in the study had social work services, most of the families were not aware of their availability and had not been referred to them. Implications that seem clear are: (1) Not only will cardiac patients require help with their anxiety, their families will as well. (2) Social service departments will have to make their services better known to patients and their families and also educate physicians about referrals.

On the premise that open-heart surgery constitutes a crisis for patients and their families, Brown and associates[9] initiated one-session educational support groups to deal with questions of discharge and posthospital recovery. The groups are jointly led by the social worker in the cardiovascular section and a nurse specialist. Patient and family groups meet separately, since their concerns just prior to discharge are not necessarily the same. Patient groups are generally preoccupied with separation from the hospital. Recognition that other patients have similar fears tends to reduce anxiety. The group members help and support one another in seeking solutions to concerns they will face after discharge. The family groups are concerned with how they can cope with the patient's emotional lability. Further, they deal with problems that the patient's behavior will have on family relationships. Evaluation of the program by patients, relatives, nurses, and physicians has been highly positive.

After observing that five of seven patients transferred from a coronary care unit to a regular hospital ward showed intense fear and anxiety, as well as cardiovascular complications, Klein and associates[32] made certain changes in the coronary care routine. In an effort to modify the fear associated with the decrease in attention and constant monitoring:

1. Patients were prepared in advance for transfer out of the unit.
2. Continuity of care was emphasized by having the patient's own physician follow the patient throughout his hospital and postdischarge course.
3. The same nurse followed the patient through the coronary care unit into the hospital ward. This nurse not only coordinated the total nursing care but spent as much as an hour a day with the patient, providing information about the medical condition and permitting discussion of feelings.

Seven patients who had the advantage of these new procedures showed no untoward changes after they were transferred from the coronary care unit.

Kornfield[34] recommends that health professionals spend time with patients before they are discharged from an intensive care unit to give them an opportunity to discuss some of the fear-producing experiences they have undergone. He suggests that information about postdischarge self-care should be more specific than, "You should take it easy," since some patients will deny the seriousness of their illness by becoming overactive, while others tend to be frightened and regress to chronic invalidism.

Golden and colleagues[26] report the development of group therapy for cardiac patients, which begins in the hospital and continues after discharge. The therapy team consists of a physician, a nurse clinician, and a group therapist (a social worker). In addition to helping the patient understand his or her physical condition, the goal is to reduce anxiety by encouraging expression of feelings. All patients indicated increased recognition of and better coping with tensions.

Repeatedly the research and study of the effects of treatment procedures, particularly of recent and more radical developments, reinforce the view that recognition of feelings and appropriate opportunity to discuss them reduces their danger for the patient.

### Feelings of Damage

Feelings that damage has been caused by the illness and/or the treatment are usually present whether or not they are readily verbalized by the patient. Feelings of damage as a result of disease or trauma may occur to a person's *image* of the body as well as to the actual physical self. A relatively intact body image—a core of self-perceptions about one's own body—is a necessary frame of reference for each individual, directly affecting the ways in which he or she functions and interacts with the world.[21] For men, disabling injuries or illnesses are more difficult to incorporate into the body image; disfiguring illnesses or injuries are most threatening to women.[56]

The body image can perhaps adjust more readily to slow changes, such as those occurring in rheumatoid arthritis with gradual stiffening of joints and loss of movement. However, traumatic changes in the aftermath of accident, amputation, or acute neurologic lesion are likely to result in more bizarre reactions (for example, the illusion of phantom limbs) and require new and painful learning by the patient.

Feelings of damage may affect the course or outcome of illness, hospitalization, and treatment. Nurses and physicians who have an understanding attitude toward their patients will anticipate these reactions and take steps to minimize the intensity and duration of such feelings. Since these feelings cannot be prevented, the focus in medical and nursing care has to be on recognition, then on constructive techniques for dealing with them.

The following examples are offered to illustrate the effects of feelings of damage and to clarify methods for coping with them:

A 75-year-old man who had enjoyed unusually good health and physical vigor as well as an active social life until his mid-sixties underwent radical surgery for the removal of a cancerous larynx. He had already survived surgery for abdominal malignancy and later the removal of an infected vocal cord. He was not informed, prior to the laryngectomy, that the surgery would deprive him of what speech he had salvaged after the loss of the vocal cord. He was told only that the present operation was necessary to save his life. During his convalescence, as he became aware of his real condition and expressed anxiety and grief, he was constantly reassured by his physician, nurses, and family that eventually he would learn to substitute esophageal for laryngeal speech. To prove his point the physician arranged a visit between the patient in the hospital and a younger man who had successfully coped with a laryngectomy by learning the new method of speech.

The patient's reaction was disappointing. He became increasingly querulous and demanding, expressing in violent gestures, fist pounding, and bed rattling what he could not express verbally. His nurses and attendants grew more and more irritable with his regression and endless bids for attention, eventually ignoring most of his bed calls. The patient gave up; his depression was obvious in his passive endurance of what was done or said to him. He was reluctant to leave his bed even when physically able. His convalescence was longer than usual for similar cases and his behavior, once he was ambulatory, became withdrawn and hostile. He used writing for essential communications.

Once home his depression and withdrawal continued. He refused to make any effort to learn available techniques of esophageal speech, avoided all social contacts, and become passively and totally dependent on his wife. At one point, in desperation, she demanded to know why he was so uncooperative. Slowly and meticulously he wrote: "Why didn't you tell me I wouldn't be a man anymore? It would have been better to die."

The lesson is clear. This patient had encompassed previous surgery and maintained contact with his world. Speech was essential to that contact. We are aware that hindsight is easier than foresight, but is it possible that this patient's sense of damage might have been mitigated by an honest appraisal of consequences with him prior to the surgery? Was the visit of a younger man who had successfully coped with a similar problem more threatening than encouraging? Was a goal established that the patient felt he could not achieve? In short, in saving this man's life, did the health team and his family demolish what remained of his self-concept and identity?

Consider in contrast the case of a young, attractive, married woman who suffers facial disfigurement in an automobile accident. Following emergency care, the surgeon talks with her husband. The doctor learns that the young wife has valued her physical appearance and has invested considerable time and care in maintaining her attractiveness. The husband is realistically appraised of the limitations of plastic surgery. He expresses more concern for his wife's well-being than her appearance. As the young women recovers, still bandaged, she is gradually and understandingly told of her condition. Her husband, who has had the opportunity to express his own grief and has been prepared for his wife's inevitable reaction to damage, is ready to comfort and support her through her struggle to accept a new body image. Her acceptance is slow. However, through the ordeal of plastic surgery and growing awareness that her appearance will not be as it was, her anguish is given free rein, her search for accommodation to her tragedy is encouraged, and her eventual shift in values is supported. She is not given unrealistic hope or palliative reassurance. Instead, with each feeble effort to reappraise her body image and seek another self-respecting role, she consistently is accepted and helped to move forward toward an altered, but still meaningful, life. She returns home subdued but ready to assume her responsibilities and live a reasonably normal life.

Again the message is obvious. In neither case could the physician, no matter how skilled, change the basic physiologic condition of his patient. However, in the first example the patient's reactions to his feelings of damage were not considered—with predictable consequences. In the second, an accepting and understanding approach contributed to a viable recovery.

Feelings of damage are also caused by certain treatment procedures, notably surgery, and especially mutilating surgery. Blacher and Basch[7] report that patients who have had pacemaker implantations say that they feel different from their former selves as well as from others. One of their patients described himself as "damaged goods." Patients who have had ileostomies and colostomies indicate a strong sense of damage. Since these procedures in their present form are unlikely to change very much and are necessary to preserve life, specific attention to the patient's feelings is an ongoing responsibility. The awareness of these potential reactions should alert the health professional to provide for open and honest discussion with patients.

The value of preparation for major surgery was clearly demonstrated by a group of anesthetists[19] who told one group of patients what to expect after surgery, taught them how to relax and how to remain more comfortable. These patients required half the postoperative narcotics for relief of pain as compared with a control group. Further, the patients who were instructed by the anesthetists were considered ready for discharge almost three days before the control group.

Another group of anesthetists[58] studied 40 patients, matched for age and levels of preoperative anxiety. One group received cursory visits from the anesthetist, while the other group received supportive visits. In the cursory interview, the patient was given a bare outline of the surgical procedure to be undergone and brief answers to questions. The anesthetist was polite, but formal. The visit lasted five minutes. The supportive interview provided the patient with all the information wanted. The anesthetist attempted to establish maximum rapport with the patient. The interview lasted as long as thirty minutes. As expected, the supportive interview reduced significantly the postsurgery anxiety level. The surprising finding was that for those who received cursory visits, the low-anxiety subgroup had a significantly higher level of anxiety immediately after surgery than did the high-anxiety subgroup.

Roy,[48] in his review of the literature, finds that appropriate preoperative intervention can lead to higher tolerance of pain and reduction of pain medications, greater acceptance of and cooperation with postoperative treatment, earlier ambulation, and earlier discharge from the hospital.

### Frustration Caused by Loss of Habitual Gratification and Pleasure

Senescu[50] has described the functions of pleasure as adaptive, buffering, nourishing, and integrative. Pleasure serves to make the stress of daily living more tolerable and has a reward effect that is stimulating and enhancing for personality growth. It may also serve to integrate and pull together various aspects of experience and personality. In this sense pleasure is neither self-indulgent nor trivial. It has wholesome significance in the individual's sense of well-being.

Illness and hospitalization inevitably interfere with daily pursuits that are rewarding and enjoyable. Whether or not confined to bed, the patient is immersed immediately in a routine of activities and services that preclude many of the usual sources of pleasure and gratification.

Clearly, the hospitalized patient does not *have* to forgo all pleasures. It is not uncommon in outpatient care for physician and patient to review what effect illness will have on certain pleasurable activities—eg, the pursuit of sports in patients with cardiac conditions. In inpatient care the stereotype of the inert, immobilized, passive patient is no longer equated with sound medical practice for all hospitalizations. Activity is recommended relatively soon after surgery or childbirth. It is not too great a move from muscular activity to pleasurable activity as a concomitant to recuperation. This shift in the concept of hospital care for certain conditions suggests that hospital personnel can learn what kinds of pleasurable activities are important for particular patients and then determine the extent to which these gratifications are feasible within the context of physical illness and hospitalization.

Some hospitals are experimenting with "minimal-care units" for ambulatory patients who are receiving diagnostic study or are convalescing. One such unit, jokingly referred to as "the Hilton," has a dayroom that allows patients a choice of recreational activities when not actually undergoing medical examination or treatment—reading, card playing, television viewing, visiting, etc. Routines (temperatures, medications, etc) are administered flexibly, patients being asked to assume the responsibility for going to the nurse's station for these services at an appropriate time. The atmosphere is relaxed, hospital personnel are not unduly burdened, and patients accept even prolonged, unpleasant, or painful examinations with a good grace. The success of "the Hilton" suggests that, with necessary modification for degrees of illness, a similar plan might be feasible in other areas of the hospital, benefiting both personnel and patients. Curiously enough, no research has been done on this matter, but it would be practical to test hypotheses concerning the relationship of pleasurable activities to prognosis and the course of illness, especially in long-term hospitalized patients.

Most treatment procedures lead to temporary loss of gratification and pleasure, easily tolerated in view of its short duration. However, in certain illnesses, treatment involves long-term or permanent changes in accustomed habits and sources of pleasure. Renal dialysis patients, as one example, are burdened with strict dietary restrictions, leading to a loss of whatever gratification was associated with eating. Male patients on dialysis suffer severe limitations in their capacity to compete at work and in athletic activities.[35,60] Halper[27] indicates that many simply "exist" on dialysis while awaiting a kidney transplant, which may be delayed for long periods of time or never materialize. Aware that withdrawal increases vulnerability to depression, Shapiro and Porush[52] arranged a seven-day, staff-organized cruise for ten dialysis patients. During the cruise, the ship's infirmary was converted to a four-bed dialysis unit. Similarly, a dialysis unit has been established at a summer camp, permitting children on dialysis to participate in all camp activities.[45] The Veterans Administration Medical Center at Iowa City[47] has arranged for guest dialysis in areas where the patient may wish to vacation.

The health professional who is aware of the deprivations imposed by treatment procedures is in a good position to assist the patient in either tolerating the loss of gratification or finding substitute sources of pleasure.

## Reactions Determined Primarily by Life Experience Prior to or During Illness

Each patient brings to illness not only a background of emotional reactions to previous illnesses but a pattern of behaving and coping developed over a lifetime. Generally, behavior under stress can be expected to be less well controlled than when the person is well. Variation in expression of feeling from patient to patient is readily observed and must be understood and, if possible, anticipated in terms of individual characteristics and life-style. It is no exaggeration to say that any person is emotionally vulnerable under the impact of serious illness. If the current sickness is complicated by a history of difficult or destructive life experiences, or capacity for coping is limited, the patient is that much more vulnerable.

Anger, dependency, and guilt are major emotional expressions that accompany physical illness and treatment. These feelings become of concern to the professional when they initiate or complicate problems of necessary patient management.

### Anger

Anger is a common and understandable reaction to frustration. It is important to distinguish *feelings* of anger from their *manifestations* in behavior, which can be explosive or destructive. A verbal expression of anger is one thing, a shouting, rampaging patient is another. Both expressions need understanding and attention, but the more manifest will demand immediate action. Beyond the obvious need to control destructiveness, however, the cause of the anger will be important to the health professional. As a result of discussion with a patient, clarification may be achieved that can effect change in the patient's feeling and possibly in the procedures to which the patient is subjected.

Anger can be not only destructive but often contagious and disruptive. Verbal expression, if accepted and understood, is usually cathartic, but explosions or tirades upset everyone involved. It is preferable to forestall violent outbursts by recognizing warning signals and intervening in the spiraling process by allowing, even encouraging, discussion of the causative frustration. When prevention is impossible, limits must be enforced that deter the patient from behavior that may harm him- or herself or others, later followed by working through the anger.

Accepting the verbalized anger and providing relevant information are two methods of handling it. Perhaps the most important concept for the health professional is to avoid responding to the angry outburst as a personal affront and answering in kind. The anger is a symptom of the patient's condition and must be treated as such with as much perspective and compassion as possible.

A nurse reported the following incident to us: As she approached a young man who was recuperating from surgery for an ulcer, he made a violent gesture in an attempt to knock the medication she was offering out of her hand. She retreated in time and somehow managed to maintain her poise as he shouted at her, "Damm you, I don't want it. It doesn't help." She had been aware that he had been restless and dissatisfied for several days. She now verbalized her awareness: "You've really been having a rough time." He responded belligerently: "You bet. Pain, pain, pain! Medicine, medicine, medicine—and still pain, pain, pain!" The nurse replied: "You mean you've had no relief?" Patient, sarcastically: –'Sure. For 10 minutes. Then I can ring the buzzer for an hour and no one comes." The nurse agreed that this was not as it should be and made the suggestion that another medication might be more effective. She volunteered to ask the physician about the matter during evening rounds. The patient was still bitter: "Sure, *you* ask him. When he comes in here, he has 10 students with him. He asks me how I feel, but before I can answer, he's showing them the incision and telling them my story—how I neglected my ulcer until I had to have an operation—and all that." The nurse: "As though you were Exhibit A instead of Don Thompson who's going through 'all that'?" He nodded, turned his head away in embarrassment, since he was now close to tears. In a few moments he went on: "My wife hasn't been to see me in three days. Calls and says she has to work second shift and is too busy during the day taking care of the kids and house. As though I'm lying here doing nothing and she has all the work to do!" The nurse now understood that this patient's symptoms of pain and anger were more complex than a simple change in medication would resolve. Since she had to continue her rounds, she said: "You've got a lot on your mind. Shall I come back later?" He nodded and now accepted the medication she silently offered again. She closed the door quietly as she left, thereby letting the patient know that she saw his need for privacy—and tears. She later took the opportunity, in a brief talk at the nurse's station with the physician, to explain tactfully the patient's upset. By the time she returned to his room, the physician had seen the patient, talked with him, and written a new drug order. The nurse reopened the interrupted discussion: "You were saying that your wife hasn't been able to visit?" He continued then with an account of family problems over a period of several years that preceded the exacerbation of his ulcer: a child's illness, financial troubles, a change of job that proved unsatisfactory, his wife's return to work, etc. No solution was reached in this one talk, but the nurse established the basis for an ongoing contact that could prove fruitful. The angry outburst became intelligible, as well as the preceding "neglect" of his ulcer. Had the nurse lost her self-possession and responded with her own anger, the results are readily imaginable.

## Dependency

Since we were all helpless infants once, residues of our dependency are the universal heritage from childhood. The extent to which dependency was acknowledged and satisfied in early childhood determines the existence and scope of the adult problem. The child whose dependency was frustrated by rejecting parents or whose early independent behavior was smothered by parental anxiety becomes an adult whose needs will be exaggerated, particularly under the stress of illness and hospitalization. An adult who has experienced independence and rewards for personal initiative and responsibility will react differently to incapacitation than will the adult who has been sheltered or denied decision making and personal control over his or her own life.

In the case of the ill, too much or too little dependency can be a complicating factor. The overly dependent patient may unconsciously look upon illness as a means of gratifying dependency wishes and may make continuous bids for attention, service, and care. Other patients will express dependency by a chronic inability to follow instructions or undertake even minimal responsibility for self-care. They will tend passively to resist encouragement to do things for themselves.

On the other hand, patients who refuse to accept the necessary dependency of illness will want to substitute their own decisions for the physician's orders. They will tend to use their own judgment of the state of their health as the guideline for their actions, and will want to discontinue medication or even leave the hospital before they are ready to do so. It is often difficult to discern from the overt behavior whether impatience with the required care stems from genuine independence or represents inner conflict about the underlying wish to be dependent. In either instance, there is a problem for medical and nursing personnel.

Hospital personnel may easily be trapped into personal rather than professional responses by the various guises of a patient's dependency. The patient may provoke behavior that fosters, denies, or attacks the dependency. The physician who becomes paternal and authoritarian may successfully meet dependency needs but may be doing so at the expense of the patient's potential for self-care. The nurse who becomes angry at a patient for basking in the attentions of others and says in exasperation, "When are you going to do something for yourself?" may stimulate anxiety, guilt, or anger. The health professional who ignores bids for attention and the dependency they imply has failed to deal with an emotional reaction, thereby unnecessarily complicating treatment procedures and the patient's prognosis.

Whenever inappropriate dependency signs are observed, these indications should become the basis for intervention by the physician or nurse. In the long run it is not helpful to gloss over this behavior and deny its presence. Dealing with the dependency need not be rejecting. Instead it can encourage at least small steps toward growth.

Illness traditionally elicits sympathy in our culture. During the course of hospitalization, there is a time when the patient who is seriously ill is naturally dependent upon the staff. However, when functioning begins to improve, too much assistance can retard the recovery process.

The following exchange between a nurse and her patient is an example of wise handling of a patient's excessive dependency:

NURSE:
Here is your lunch tray, Mr. A.

PATIENT:
Aren't you going to feed me today?

NURSE:
No, it is important that you begin using that arm.

PATIENT (pouting):
All right, I won't eat, then.

NURSE:
I'll be back in a half hour for the tray.

The nurse returns as she promised. The food remains untouched. She takes the tray away without comment. She is not angry or belittling but simply matter-of-fact. The patient understands that she meant what she said. He feeds himself dinner, awkwardly and painfully, but successfully. By not succumbing to the patient's bid for continued dependency, the nurse has lessened the possibility of a prolonged recovery or even a chronic convalescence.

It is not easy to forgo our desire to provide immediate help for the patient. The staff of any hospital have strong needs for serving others. The endless doing for patients is part of the routine that gives meaning to many hospital positions. Much of the intangible reward for working in a hospital is the belief that the little things done for patients help their comfort, well-being, and eventual recuperation. For these reasons, it is often difficult to interrupt the cycle of responding to requests for service, especially services that were necessary at one point in the course of illness. It is quite possible, however, for hospital personnel to distinguish between real needs for service and those demands or wishes that signify other needs (for attention, recognition, etc). In serving the patient, essential well-being rather than immediate demands should be the criterion.

### Guilt

The causes and manifestations of guilt are even more subtle and complex than fear or anger and therefore can be more insidious and difficult to handle. Perhaps the most frequent reason for guilt over incapacitation lies in our moral concepts of role responsibility. A male head-of-family breadwinner may suffer guilt because he is not working and earning his salary, whether or not his income has actually ceased as a result of illness. This feeling is tied to our association of masculinity with providing responsibly for one's family. Women who do not work outside the home often find their activities of managing a home and family equivalent responsibilities that lead to their concept of a good wife and mother. To be removed from the home for reasons they cannot control becomes a source of guilt.

Guilt may also arise from conditions other than restrictions on the normal role functions that lend stability and meaning to individual life. Guilt may occur when illness is viewed as punishment. It may also be a reaction to anger against the "healthy ones," family members and others who remain intact and undamaged by physical illness.

The person who experiences guilt may withdraw into passive tolerance of pain and disability, communicating only tersely and ineffectively with the physician and nurses, or at the other extreme, may project this guilt as blame and be fault-finding, quarrelsome, and chronically dissatisfied with the hospital or the treatment provided.

Whenever a patient is withdrawn, it is important to discover if this retreat is a preoccupation based on guilt. Guilt that is allowed to fester may become depression. Senescu[50] recommends exploring any unexplained withdrawal by a direct inquiry concerning possible guilt.

Generally speaking, while the effects of guilt may be genuinely debilitating and may complicate treatment procedures, sources of guilt usually are unreal; that is, they derive from distorted perceptions of persons, circumstances, and values.

An ex-army sergeant in his thirties requested admission to his local Veterans Administration Medical Center for treatment of stomach pain and associated symptoms. His condition seemed to warrant further study and therefore he was admitted. However, thorough examination, laboratory tests, and x-rays did not reveal a physiologic basis for his pain, his inability to retain food, and his diarrhea. When an inquiry was made about his life situation, he told of the recent birth of a defective child—a hydrocephalic boy—who was still in the hospital. The patient and his wife had made daily trips of 40 miles each way to visit the hospital to see the child and receive reports of progress. It was suggested that doubts about the child's survival might be of concern to him. His denial was emphatic. He stated that he and his wife had resolved this problem; they could accept the possibility of death, but, should the child live, they would do their best to care for him. He insisted that the only problem was his stomach complaint that kept him from returning to work. If he did not work, he received no salary, and hospital bills for the child were mounting. The cost of the child's hospitalization was of particular concern since he had no hospital insurance. Exploration then centered on his feelings about having to care for a defective child if that child should live. Although he claimed to be unconcerned about that likelihood, he added, "Maybe you'd better ask my wife about that. She'd be taking care of him most of the time." The patient and his wife were interviewed together on her next visit to the hospital. During this interview, the wife revealed that the child had been conceived four months before the marriage. The patient looked angrily at her, then hung his head in shame and said, "That's what's bothering me. That child is our punishment for doing something against my religion. I haven't even been able to tell the priest about it." Several more sessions were held with the patient and his wife, encouraging discussion about what they described as "our sin." His symptoms were relieved sufficiently so that he was able to return home and to work. Counseling sessions continued for several months, helping this couple to work through their distress, shame, and fear of caring for a defective child. The husband remained free of his previously disabling complaints.

It is significant that each advance in medical and surgical treatment, dramatically lifesaving as it may be, cannot escape the complication of emotional distress. The miracle of transplants, for example, is often dimmed in the aftermath of the patient's reaction to what has happened. Recipients of kidneys seem particularly vulnerable to sometimes disabling guilt. They often feel that others have suffered because of their illness. Severe guilt is experienced by those who receive the organ of a living donor as well as those who have transplants from recently deceased persons. In the first case, the patients fear that the living donor may die; in the second, that they may have been in some way responsible for the donor's death.[31] Abram[1] describes a patient who became severely depressed upon realizing that in his hope for a transplant he had really wished for the death of another person. Muslin[43] describes guilt in recipients of cadaver kidneys over being unable to pay back or having taken something for nothing.

An important reason for recognizing, accepting, and understanding guilt reactions is to prevent more serious consequences in depression. In several instances, rewarding results have been reported through the use of therapeutic intervention. For example, in one program a team of nurse clinician and social worker,[55] in another of psychiatrist and gynecologist[11] reported success with group therapy to relieve the guilt of women who have undergone therapeutic abortions.

## Reactions of Depression and Loss of Self-Esteem to Illness and Treatment

Whenever immediate symptoms of personal distress are not relieved by the methods described above, there is the possibility that the more dangerous emotional reactions of depression and loss of self-esteem will occur.

### Depression
Although the behavior associated with depression usually follows a recognizable pattern (withdrawal, dejection, unwillingness to talk, eat, or engage in activity), it is important to distinguish between the depression that is a reaction to hospitalization and illness (reactive depression) and that which is more long-standing in the patient's history. Reactive depression is characterized by a relatively sudden onset, a generalized slowing down, and a constant feeling of sadness. Self-control is maintained, as is the ability to make important decisions. Usually there is enough energy for brief periods of apparent recovery. However, depression that has roots in the patient's previous life experience is evidenced by greater fluctuations in mood and self-esteem, with more intense expressions of fear concerning the present and the future. Poor concentration may interfere with decision making. An impaired sense of responsibility and frequent distortions of events are also characteristic. Relationships with hospital personnel and family members are generally poor, fluctuating, and laden with anger, fear, and anxiety.

Reactive depression has a situational origin: the patient's physical condition and hospitalized status. Physicians and nurses should try to deal with this depression (1) by being aware that it does in fact exist, and (2) by a direct assessment with the patient of the reality of this reaction. In most instances, both the intensity and the duration of depression can be reduced in this manner.[36] (For an illustration of the effective handling of a reactive depression, the reader might wish to review the nurse's interview with Mrs. Carson in Chapter 5.) However, when a depression is judged to be more deeply rooted and does not respond readily, a referral may need to be made to a specialist in emotional disturbances.

Depression is the second most frequently reported reaction to some of the newer treatment techniques (anxiety being the first). Depression as a reaction to the multiple frustrations of renal dialysis, for example, is indeed understandable. The decision of some patients to discontinue living on chronic hemodialysis appears related to decreased hope, as the expectation of a transplant remains unfulfilled.[23] In this connection McKegney and Lange[38] state: "The reaction might be analogous to that of a child's, if every night were Christmas Eve but every morning just another day, not Christmas" (p. 271). They recommend discussing, at the beginning of the dialysis program, the possibility of withdrawal if a life of constant dependency on a machine and perpetual physical discomfort should become too difficult. Although such an approach may seem discouraging from the start, it can serve as a realistic point of reference if the patient feels free to discuss this matter with the staff at a later date. Since there is reliable evidence that talking about suicidal intentions decreases rather than increases the likelihood that suicide will occur, open discussion about withdrawal from dialysis may be expected to have a similar effect.

Halper[27] feels that the potential for suicide should be evaluated in dialysis patients who develop even moderately severe depressions. He recommends encouraging free expression of their feelings of depression, pointing out that patients usually will respond to comments from health professionals such as, "It sounds that at times you've considered ending it all."

Living donors of kidneys for transplant may also experience feelings of rejection and depression after the expressions of gratitude have waned and attention is once again directed to the recipient.[16]

If the body rejects the transplanted kidney, the patient will need to return to chronic dialysis. These patients tend to experience relief initially at coming back to a familiar environment and a predictable life. However, in spite of this sense of relief, the dialysis staff may expect reactions of rage, depression, and feelings of loss over the unsuccessful transplant by the patient and family. Carosella[12] suggests that, although the dialysis nurses may be tempted to join the patient in projecting anger onto the transplant team, they can best serve the patient and family by creating a safe environment for the expression of their feelings.

Winkelstein and Lyons[59] have found depression to be an almost inevitable reaction of patients with ileostomies and colostomies, who are suddenly deprived of bowel control. Because great importance is placed on the control of excretions, the loss of control of these functions is difficult to tolerate. Members of ostomy societies, who function in a manner similar to Alcoholics Anonymous, visit patients in and after discharge from the hospital. The value of these visits appears to be in the patient's realization that he or she is not alone and that others have adjusted to the stoma.

Cassem and Hackett[13] surveyed all patients admitted to the coronary-care unit of the Massachusetts General Hospital during a 15-month period. Of the 445 admissions to the unit, one third were referred for psychiatric consultation, primarily for anxiety and depression. They found that early physical mobilization soon after recovery begins is a most useful method of combating these psychiatric symptoms. Although the physical weakness experienced upon returning home is due to muscle atrophy and the systemic effects of immobilization, these patients tend to attribute it to heart damage. Consequently, the early mobilization counteracts both the physical and psychologic consequences of immobilization. Psychologically, it gives the patient something to *do* in a regimen which consists largely of *don'ts*.

Depression has been found to be the chief deterrent to rehabilitation of patients with maxillofacial cancers.[49] The Maxillofacial Rehabilitation Clinic of the University of California School of Dentistry is using individual and group psychotherapy, speech therapy, and supportive environmental resources in an effort to overcome the depression so often noted in these patients. In addition, the services of a vocational counselor are available to assist the patient to return to his or her former type of work or to enter retraining programs.

Women whose biologic functions are modified by medication or surgery seem highly prone to depression, perhaps because these functions are intimately related to psychologic well-being. In a study of 70 women on oral contraceptives who had no previous history of psychiatric illness, the major psychologic side effect was depression with associated loss of libidinal interest. These side effects were related to ambivalence about having more children, rather than a firm decision to avoid pregnancy. The investigaors[22] recommend that physicians should determine with each patient whether she really wants a contraceptive or is accommodating to certain pressures—her husband's wish to limit the family, economic considerations, or social disapproval. Emotional disturbances and marital or sexual problems should be evaluated. It was found that maladjusted women on the "pill" were more likely to report side effects than those of good emotional adjustment. In other words, the ready availability of contraceptives should not be the only determinant for their use.

Depression has also been found to be the most common emotional reaction to hysterectomy.[46] Barker[3] compared 729 hysterectomized women with 280 who had had cholecystomies during the same period of time. There was a two-and-one-half times higher frequency of psychiatric referral for those who had undergone hysterectomies; the referral rate was approximately three times higher than the expected incidence for women of the same age in the general population. Where marital problems were present, there was a six times greater frequency of psychiatric referral after hysterectomy as compared with those who had stable marriages. Chafetz[14] suggests that physicians take the time to discuss the emotional problems of hysterectomy at the time the decision is made for the operation as a means of lowering the postoperative complications.

Keith[30] reports on the success of posthysterectomy discussion groups, with a social worker and a nurse serving as leaders. The nurse provides technical information and the social worker focuses on emotional and psychosocial matters.

Similar findings have been reported for women who have had mastectomies. In a review of six recent controlled studies of mastectomy, Miller[40] reports that many of these women, as well as their husbands, suffered from depression, anxiety, suicidal thoughts, sexual problems, lowered self-esteem, and family adjustment problems. It was also reported that a healthier postmastectomy adjustment was made by those who received information, education, support, and counseling.

Verwoerdt points out that a vague ill-defined depression is likely to be among the earliest symptoms of diseases with widespread systemic effects (eg, carcinoma of the pancreas). He suggests that early systemic disease be suspected in those cases in which the patient complains of depression, especially when there has been no previous history of depressive illness.[56]

### Loss of Self-esteem
Self-esteem derives from a conglomerate of values, attitudes, and assumptions about oneself that determine the level of self-regard. For relatively well-functioning persons, this level of self-regard fluctuates only slightly in response to external events, to internal psychologic

states, or to physiologic conditions. Adequate self-regard enables an integration of judgment and decision making so that realistic appraisal of life circumstances and events is possible.

In prolonged illness with ensuing dependency, self-esteem is severely taxed. Loss of self-esteem usually is manifested in reduced cooperation with treatment procedures. More subtle is the minimization of the patient's perception of improvement. As a result the patient is likely to give hospital personnel an inaccurate and negative account of the condition, thereby predisposing them against perceiving improvement. It is only one step from those distorted perceptions to genuine retardation of healing processes. The patient accepts illness, defeat, and institutionalization instead of actively participating in the treatment process.

Low self-esteem is not independent of depression. Since signals of depression are much more visible than cues for impaired self-regard, there tends to be greater awareness of depression. However, patients who suffer from longstanding depression also, by definition, have had their self-esteem impoverished and undermined. The patient who responds to hospitalization with reactive depression may maintain a more intact self-regard, but the fluctuations will be greater than usual and positive feelings about the self will be more fragile and less consistent.

Expressions of anger, dependency, or guilt should be handled as soon as they are recognized. Otherwise the professional may have to contend with the more pervasive and disruptive effects of depression and reduced self-esteem.


## THE EFFECTS OF FAMILY RELATIONS ON ILLNESS

The importance of the family in health and illness has already been discussed in Chapter 1 (section on the family practice specialty) and Chapter 8 ("Interviewing the Family"). There is little doubt that the attitude of the family toward its sick member can markedly influence the patient's response to both illness and treatment.

If evidence is needed, the literature abounds in studies and reports to support this view. For example, one investigation[10] demonstrates that strongly supportive family relationships play a part in preventing the more devastating effects of illness when it occurs. A study of coronary heart disease was carried out in two neighboring communities in Pennsylvania. One community had a significantly higher death rate from myocardial infarction than the other. There were no differences in the physical findings between the cardiac patients in these two communities that could account for the difference in the death rate. What was markedly different was the nature of family and social life in the two communities. In the town with the lower death rate, the population, Italian-Americans in the lower socioeconomic range, adhered to the religious traditions and dietary customs of their ethnic background. Families, nuclear and extended, were closely knit, mutually supportive, and gregarious. In contrast, the town with the higher death rate was a lower-middle-class community of mixed ethnic background: English, Welsh, German, Italian. Independence and self-sufficiency were valued, rather than strong family life, and distinctive community customs and traditions were lacking.

If supportive family behavior has a clearly positive effect on health, family indifference or hostility is just as effective in a negative, damaging sense. Some families resist accepting a member in the sick role and continue to function as if the symptoms are quite normal. Later, if hospitalization becomes necessary, guilt may lead to excessive concern and attention, delaying the patient's recovery. Or when the period of hospitalization is lengthy, the family may reorganize itself to fill the gap left by the patient. Then if the new pattern of relationships functions well, the patient's eventual return is disruptive and therefore resented.[56]

Malmquist[37] found that dialysis patients whose spouses were rated as anxious demonstrated greater anxiety themselves than patients with relatively nonanxious mates. Similarly, Moore,[41] who studied patients in the Mayo Clinic's dialysis program over a two-year period, found that one major factor that discriminated between the patients who adjusted more successfully rather than less successfully was the presence of a supportive family.

Since these findings seem so self-evident, it is indeed surprising that the family is so often ignored in medical practice. In their well-known investigation, Duff and Hollingshead[18] studied over 200 families in which one member had been admitted to the hospital. In 47 percent of the cases, there was clear evidence that the illness was linked to unsatisfactory family relationships. Yet only about one-third of the physicians had any awareness of these relationships; only 21 percent of the doctors were fully aware of the associated family problem, 15 percent were partially aware, and 64 percent were totally unaware.

The health professional who understands this matter will make it a point to include family members in important decisions about the patient's treatment and self-care. He or she will be alert to changing attitudes toward the patient and use these observations in working with the family.

## PSYCHOLOGIC INTERVENTION

Throughout this chapter we have referred to a variety of interventions intended to deal with the emotional factors related to illness and treatment. In a classic study, Mumford and her associates[42] analyzed the outcomes of all the studies they could locate that examined the effects of psychologic intervention on preoperative patients or patients recovering from heart attack. They found 34 published and unpublished controlled experimental studies, carried out between 1955 and 1978. Using meta-analysis (a statistical technique that permits one to determine the effects of intervention across many different investigations), they found that for 210 different outcome measures, the intervention groups were superior to the control groups. Only 15 percent of the 210 outcome indicators were negative. Among the outcomes with the highest ratings were: cooperation with treatment, speed of recovery, and fewer postdischarge complications.

The interventions were categorized as educational (providing patients with information) and psychologic (emotional support). Although psychologic methods were somewhat more effective than the educational, a combination of the two methods was clearly superior to either one alone. Further, the length of hospital stay was reduced by approximately two days for the intervention groups.

These investigators conclude their findings with the following statement:

> It is often argued that the medical care system cannot afford to take on the emotional status of the patient as its responsibility. Time is short and costs are high. However, it may be that medicine cannot afford to ignore the patient's emotional status assuming that it will take care of itself. Anxiety and depression do not go away by being ignored. The psychological and physiological expressions of emotional upheaval may be themselves disastrous for the delicately balanced patient or may lead to behavior that needlessly impedes recovery when surgery or medical treatment was otherwise successful.
>
> Usually advances in medical knowledge call for large investments in training, personnel, and equipment if patients are to benefit. Thus, a measure that promises to benefit pa-

tients and to save money at the same time is newsworthy (p. 144).

A member of the editorial board[57] of the journal in which the above study appeared was prompted to write an editorial comment as follows:

In their article, "The Effects of Psychological Intervention on Recovery from Surgery and Heart Attacks: An Analysis of the Literature," published in this issue of the Journal, Mumford, Schlesinger, and Glass have made an important contribution to our understanding regarding the role of interpersonal skills in medical and surgical care. Most residency training programs have been designed so that knowing when and how to perform a procedure or which medicine to prescribe are adequate abilities. Skills in communicating with patients have generally been viewed as necessary, but unimportant or placebo aspects of patient care which are learned through experience. As the "art" of medicine, such techniques cannot be scheduled nor taught, or so the stereotype goes; and they have no particular influence on patient outcomes. This careful review article sheds serious doubts on such notions.

The authors have drawn on a widely distributed literature for their review. Reports came from journals which serve primary care physicians, pediatricians, internists, surgeons, psychiatrists, immunologists, dentists, nurses, psychologists, and medical social scientists. The isolation of these investigators in a variety of fields has probably impeded their influence on medical and surgical practice.

Another valuable contribution by the authors has been to subdivide the general area of interpersonal skills management into: (1) education and (2) one-to-one interactions, such as discussion regarding the patient's questions and concerns—sometimes referred to as counseling or (in mental health jargon) supportive psychotherapy. Lumping all interpersonal skills into one broad category serves only to obfuscate the complex issues involved. It is of interest that the data support the utility of applying both approaches, rather than employing just education or just a psychotherapeutic modality.

What are the implications of these findings for the health field? First, we must be much more concerned about training health professionals in interpersonal skills, such as education, counseling, and relaxation techniques. This is especially true for those fields in which the primary emphasis has been on the acquisition of biomedical information and technical skills. These disciplines include dentists, most physicians and surgeons, and many nurses. This is not to say that these professional groups must become "compleat" psychotherapists; however, they must be able to educate and counsel patients about the medical interventions and technical procedures which they perform. Merely exposing students and trainees to experienced clinicians does not guarantee either that they will acquire interpersonal skills adequate to their tasks, or that they will understand the importance of such skills on patient outcomes. In this regard, the National Board of Medical Examiners has recently established an Interpersonal Skills Task Force to generate test items which address this important area. It appears that, at least at the level of certification and licensure, there is growing awareness regarding the importance of these skills for professional competence.

An important corollary issue involves the assignment of clinical responsibility for interpersonal skills in health services. It seems likely that in time both consumers as well as administrators of health services will recognize the importance of such transactions to patient outcomes. If health professionals do not discharge these responsibilities during their provision of services, it seems likely that others will be hired and trained to meet them. This can only add to the cost of medical care, as well as to the fragmentation and depersonalization of health services.

Another implication of this report concerns economics. The authors have demonstrated that the provision of education and brief psychotherapies tended to reduce cost, while also reducing morbidity and mortality. Yet, the recent trend in health care insurance has been to reduce or refuse recompense for such services. It is not likely that a fee submitted by a physician or surgeon for counseling or education would be honored, nor that a hospital administrator would permit nursing time to be devoted to similar endeavors. Thus, our current economic, political, and administrative structures obstruct the implementation of these findings.

As with most innovative studies, these findings raise new issues for us. In particular, further attention should be paid to the minority (15 percent) of the findings which do not support the hypothesis. As the authors indicate, we should not assume that education and counseling are necessarily good for everyone despite general trends. We need to know when the application of these interpersonal skills is either unnecessary or even counterproductive. So-called Hawthorne effects, stemming from such nonspecific factors as increased staff–patient interactions, may account for much or all of the observed differences. There remains the possibility that other data supporting the null hypothesis have not been published, given the difficulty in publishing such reports.

Many humanistic and/or experienced clinicians will view these data as merely explicating the obvious. For many others involved in the provision of health services, the results are not so obvious. As the Chinese-American medical anthropologist Francis Hsu has observed, "The Chinese accept science if it is clothed as magic, while Americans accept magic if it is clothed as science." Many health practitioners view the application of interpersonal skills in clinical interactions as evidencing more of the magic of medicine rather than its skillful and scientific application. We need such studies as these to provide enlightened and effective health services which are both humanistic and scientific.

Joseph Westermeyer, MD, MPH, PhD (pp. 126–7)

## EFFECTS OF POSITIVE EMOTIONS ON ILLNESS

In concluding this chapter on the role of emotion in illness and treatment, we wish to bring to attention a most welcome positive note recently sounded in the discussion of this subject. While the negative effects of negative emotion—fear, anxiety, anger, depression, etc—have been studied extensively, there has been less documentation of the positive effects of positive emotion—a strong will to live because life itself is highly valued, a determination to go on because of happy family and social relationships and a joy in work, a sense of one's capacity to understand and master the threat to one's life.

Several persons of prominence and distinction, having suffered usually life-threatening illness, have lately made public their personal struggles to overcome their disease. Among them is Susan Sontag, who, in a television interview, recounted her remarkable success in recovering from cancer. Understanding just how deadly the threat was, she used her high intelligence to learn everything she could about her illness. She became more knowledgeable than many physicians and was therefore in a strong position to act in her own behalf, change doctors, and seek out reliable treatment (not quackery) that seemed to offer hope. Her intellectual and probably financial resources are, of course, unusual, but her point that passive acceptance of medical diagnoses and decisions is neither necessary nor universally expected by physicians could serve as an encouraging model.

In another account, Abram,[2] a New York City attorney of outstanding achievement, writes ". . . a compelling personal story of a rare individual who has defied odds and lived for five years in remission from acute myelocytic leukemia" (p. 3).[6] His is a moving report of personal determination and courage that has successfully prolonged his life.

Norman Cousins, the well-known former editor of the *Saturday Review,* and presently a senior lecturer in the University of California, Los Angeles, School of Medicine, has survived a coronary occlusion and ankylosing spondylitis, an arthritic-like crippling disease (which did not cripple him). He attributes his recovery, in part, to "deep belly laughter," and his report[15] has stimulated research on the effects of laughter on health. In his review of such research, Fry[25] points out that a lively sense of humor is related to healthy coping mechanisms. At the Andrus Gerontology Center in Los Angeles, it has been found that a humor "program" (puppetry, exchange of jokes and cartoons, etc) led to improved morale, activity level, and socialization among the patients. There is good reason to believe that laughter can bring about the beneficial effects of aerobic exercise (eg, increasing the vitality of the immune system, sense of well-being, pain relief) since the physiologic mechanisms of exercise and laughter are similar. Laughter may also serve to dispel fear and anger, since mirth and negative emotions cannot exist at the same time.

## SUMMARY

Emotion can be a potent force in causing illness, complicating and/or prolonging it, and reducing the effectiveness of treatment. Responsible care of patients must include recognizing, understanding, and dealing appropriately with emotional reactions if optimal benefits are to be obtained.

Physiologic reactions to emotional stress and the frequency of functional illness are well known. Yet professionals tend to pay little attention to these symptoms if a physiologic cause cannot be found. However, awareness of lack of skill and poor preparation for treating functional illness is increasing.

Recent research discloses the surprising new concept that ordinary and even favorable life events can predispose the individual to illness, if too many of these events occur too closely in time and involve changes that require an excessive amount of coping. Medical practice, based on sound relationships with patients, has a high potential for preventive care by keeping aware of expected life changes and encouraging appropriate coping methods.

Certain emotional reactions are likely to manifest themselves as a direct result of the illness or treatment: fear, feelings of damage, and frustration caused by loss of habitual gratification and pleasure.

Fear is defined as anticipatory dread of pain, danger, or disfigurement. Intense expressions of fear and anxiety sap the patient's strength and consume energy that could be more constructively used in combating the illness or in contributing to the recuperative process. When information and understanding methods do not suffice to reduce the fear, it may be necessary to confront the patient with the exaggerated fear in realistic, not hostile, terms.

Anxiety inadvertently precipitated by medical attention (iatrogenic anxiety) can be avoided by explaining treatment procedures in understandable and understanding terms. Repeatedly research and study of effects of treatment procedures, particularly recent more radical developments, reinforce the view that recognition of feelings of fear and appropriate opportunity to discuss them reduces their danger for the patient.

Feelings of damage to a person's body image as well as to the actual physical self may occur. Methods for dealing with these feelings include an accepting attitude toward the patient's behavior and feelings, encouraging a "climate" for open expression of feelings, reflecting feelings in a way that offers the patient an opportunity to consider alternatives for improvement or resolution of the problem, giving accurate and appropriate information about the physical condition and its prognosis, and providing a continuing relationship until improvement or resolution is achieved.

Illness, hospitalization, and certain treatment procedures interfere with activities that are rewarding and enjoyable. Physicians and nurses should encourage the continuation of a patient's usual sources of pleasure to the extent possible. The health professional who is aware of the deprivations imposed by illness or treatment is in a good position to assist the patient in either tolerating the loss of gratification or in finding substitute sources of pleasure.

In addition to the above triad of emotional responses directly related to the illness or treatment, the patient's other experiences prior to or during the illness will determine the extent to which other emotional factors—anger, dependency, and guilt—will complicate his or her responses.

Anger can be contagious and disruptive. It is preferable to forestall outbursts by recognizing warning signals and intervening before explosive or destructive expressions of anger occur. Giving information and accepting the anger are appropriate in handling it. It is important that the health professional not react to the anger as a personal affront or respond in kind. When prevention is not possible, limits must be enforced that deter the patient from behavior that may harm him- or herself or others, later followed by working through the anger.

The overly dependent patient may make continuous bids for attention, service, and care. There is a time during serious illness when a patient necessarily is dependent on hospital staff for existence itself. However, when functions begin to improve, too much assistance from staff can retard the recovery process.

While the effects of guilt may be genuinely debilitating and complicating for treatment procedures, sources of guilt are usually unreal; that is, they derive from distorted perceptions of persons, circumstances, and values. An important reason for recognizing, accepting, and understanding guilt reactions is to prevent more serious consequences in depression and loss of self-esteem.

Health professionals should deal with depression (1) by being aware that it does in fact exist, and (2) by direct assessment with the patient of the reality of this reaction. In most instances both the intensity and the duration of depression can be reduced by an understanding acceptance of feelings of sadness and loss of self-esteem. However, when depression is judged to be rooted more deeply and does not respond readily, psychiatric assistance may be required.

The reaction of the family to the illness of one of its members may be potentially destructive or highly supportive. Health professionals should include the family in important decisions about treatment and self-care of the patient and, when possible, use the family interview to modify negative attitudes toward the patient.

Many of the untoward effects of emotions in illness and treatment can be positively modified by intervention, which should include both educational and psychologic aspects. Among the most important outcomes of such intervention are improved cooperation with treatment, speedier recovery, and fewer postdischarge complications.

Recently a highly encouraging point of view has been expressed by several well-known persons who have overcome or learned to live effectively with life-threatening illness. They demonstrate that positive feeling and action can be as effective in overcoming illness as negative emotion can be in causing or complicating it. Their experience might well serve as models for other sick people and as an incentive for research into the effects of positive emotions.

# REFERENCES

1. Abram HS: The psychiatrist, the treatment of chronic renal failure, and the prolongation of life: III. Am J Psychiatry 128:1534, 1972
2. Abram MB: Living with leukemia. In Bernstein E (ed): Medical and Health Annual. Chicago, Encyclopaedia Britannica, 1979
3. Barker B: Psychiatric illness after hysterectomy. Br Med J 2:91, 1968
4. Beard BH: Fear of death and fear of life. Arch Gen Psychiatry 21:373, 1969
5. Bennett EA: The anxiety state. Br Med J 2:554, 1953
6. Bernstein E: Foreword. In Bernstein E (ed): Medical and Health Annual. Chicago, Encyclopaedia Britannica, 1979
7. Blacher RS, Basch SH: Psychological aspects of pacemaker implantation. Arch Gen Psychiatry 22:319, 1970
8. Branch CHH: Postgraduate psychiatric education of physicians: an overview. In Feldman R, Buck DP (eds): Eighth Annual Training Session for Psychiatrist-Teachers of Practicing Physicians—1967. Boulder, Western Interstate Commission for Higher Education, 1968
9. Brown DG, Glazer H, Higgins M: Group intervention: a psychosocial and educational approach to open heart surgery patients and their families. Social Work in Health Care 9 (2):47, 1983
10. Bruhn JG, Chandler B, Miller C, Wolf S, Lynn TN: Social aspects of coronary heart disease in two adjacent, ethnically different communities. Am J Public Health 56:1493, 1966
11. Burnell GM, Dworsky WA, Harrington RL: Post-abortion group therapy. Am J Psychiatry 129:220, 1972
12. Carosella J: Picking up the pieces: the unsuccessful kidney transplant. Health and Social Work 9:142, 1984
13. Cassem NH, Hackett TP: Psychological aspects of myocardial infarction. Med Clin North Am 61:711, 1977
14. Chafetz ME: Hysterectomy-castration: an emotional look-alike. Med Insight 3:38, 1971
15. Cousins N: Anatomy of an illness (as perceived by the patient). N Engl J Med 295:1458, 1976
16. Cramond WA: Renal transplantation—experiences with recipients and donors. Semin Psych 3:116, 1971
17. Dhooper SS: Family coping with the crisis of heart attack. Social Work in Health Care 9(1):15, 1983
18. Duff RS, Hollingshead AB: Sickness and Society. New York, Harper & Row, 1968
19. Egbert LD, Battit GE, Welch CE, Bartlett MK: Reduction of post-operative

pain by encouragement and instruction of patients: a study of doctor-patient rapport. N Engl J Med 270:825, 1964

20. Ell KO, De Guzman M, Haywood LJ: Stressful life events: a predictor in recovery from heart attacks. Health and Social Work 8:133, 1983
21. Fisher S, Cleveland SF: Body Image and Personality. Princeton, Van Nostrand, 1958
22. Fortin JN, Wittkower ED, Paiement J, Tetreault L: Side effects of oral contraceptive medication: a psychosomatic problem. Can Psychiatr Assoc J 17:3, 1972
23. Foster TA: Why patients decide to discontinue renal dialysis. J Am Med Women's Assn 31:234, 1976
24. Frank KA, Heller SS, Kornfield DS: A survey of adjustment to cardiac surgery. Arch Intern Med 130:735, 1972
25. Fry WF Jr: Laughter and health. In Bernstein E (ed): Medical and Health Annual. Chicago, Encyclopaedia Britannica, 1984
26. Golden JH, Golden NP, Dibiase J: Crisis intervention for cardiac patients. Med Insight 4:18, 1972
27. Halper IS: Psychiatric observations in a chronic hemodialysis program. Med Clin North Am 55:177, 1971
28. Holmes TH, Masuda M: Psychosomatic syndrome. Psychol Today 5:71, 1972
29. Holmes TH, Masuda M: Life change and illness susceptibility in separation and depression. In Scott JP, Senay EC (eds): Separation and Depression. Washington, DC, American Association for the Advancement of Science, pub. no. 94, 1973
30. Keith C: Discussion group for posthysterectomy patients. Health and Social Work 5:59, 1980
31. Kemph JP, Berman EA, Copolillo HP: Kidney transplant and shift in family dynamics. Am J Psychiatry 125:1485, 1969
32. Klein RF, Kliner VS, Zipes DP, Troyer WG Jr, Wallace AG: Transfer from a coronary care unit. Arch Intern Med 122:104, 1968
33. Klopfer B: Psychological variables in human cancer. J Projective Techniques 21:329, 1957
34. Kornfield DS: Psychiatric problems of an intensive care unit. Med Clin North Am 55:1353, 1971
35. MacNamara M: Psychosocial problems in a renal unit. Br J Psychiatry 113:1231, 1967
36. Mailick MD: The short-term treatment of depression of physically ill hospital patients. Social Work in Health Care 9 (3):51, 1984
37. Malmquist A: A prospective study of patients in chronic hemodialysis. I. Method and characteristics of the patient group. J Psychosom Res 17:333, 1973
38. McKegney FP, Lange P: The decision to no longer live on chronic hemodialysis. Am J Psychiatry 128:267, 1971
39. Menzel H, Coleman J, Katz E: Dimensions of being "modern" in medical practice. J Chron Dis 9:20, 1959

40. Miller PJ: Mastectomy: A review of psychosocial research. Health and Social Work 6:60, 1981
41. Moore GL: Psychiatric aspects of chronic renal dialysis. Postgrad Med 60:140, 1976
42. Mumford E, Schlesinger HJ, Glass GV: The effects of psychological intervention on recovery from surgery and heart attacks: an analysis of the literature. Am J Public Health 72:141, 1982
43. Muslin HL: The emotional response to kidney transplant: the process of internalization. Can Psychiatr Assoc J 17:SS-3, 1972
44. Petrich J, Holmes TH: Life change and onset of illness. Med Clin North Am 61:825, 1977
45. Primack WA, Melber S, Greifer I: Hemodialysis at a summer camp. Proc Clin Dialysis and Transplant Forum 4:91, 1975
46. Roeske NCA: Quality of life and factors affecting the response to hysterectomy. J Fam Pract 7:483, 1978
47. Roy C, Dowler D: Planning vacations with dialysis patients. Health and Social Work 5:61, 1980
48. Roy R: Psychological preparation for surgical patients. Health and Social Work 6:44, 1981
49. Rozen RD, Ordway DE, Curtis TA, Cantor R: Psychosocial aspects of maxillofacial rehabilitation. Part 1. The effect of primary cancer treatment. J Prosth Dentistry 28:423, 1972
50. Senescu RA: The development of emotional complications in the patient with cancer. J Chron Dis 16:813, 1963
51. Shanan J, De-Nour AK, Garty I: Effects of prolonged stress on coping style in terminal renal failure patients. J Hum Stress 2:19, 1976
52. Shapiro WB, Porush JG: Shipboard dialysis. J Dialysis 1:825, 1977
53. Smith, CK, Cullison SW, Holmes TH: Life change and illness onset: Importance of concepts for family physicians. J Fam Pract 9:975, 1978
54. Stern M, Pascale L, Ackerman A: Life adjustment postmyocardial infarction. Arch Intern Med 137:1680, 1977
55. Ullman A: Social work service to abortion patients. Social Casework 53:481, 1972
56. Verwoerdt A: Psychopathological responses to the stress of physical illness. Adv Psychosom Med 8:119, 1972
57. Westermeyer J: Education and counseling in hospital care (editorial). Am J Public Health 72:127, 1982
58. Williams JGL, Jones JR, Workman MC, Williams B: The psychological control of preoperative anxiety. Psychophysiology 12:50, 1975
59. Winkelstein C, Lyons AS: Insight into the emotional aspects of ileostomies and colostomies. Med Insight 3:15, 1971
60. Wright RG, Sand P, Livingston G: Psychological stress during hemodialysis for chronic renal failure. Ann Intern Med 3:611, 1966

# chapter 11

# Social Distance
# and Patient Care

Social distance refers to differences between the health professional and the patient, which can be a major barrier in the professional–patient interview situation. Simmons,[19] after studying the relationship between social distance and medical care, concluded that trust, respect, and cooperation in the professional–patient relationship will vary inversely with the amount of social distance. In other words, with patients of similar status, health professionals are more likely to establish a relationship of openness and responsible participation. On the other hand, the values and life-styles of patients of different status may not be understood or accepted by the middle-class practitioner. These patients do not fit the professional's concept of a "good" patient and are likely to be considered uncooperative, unpleasant, or dull. Accordingly, physicians and nurses may respond with less interest in and, inadvertently, with less attention to those patients of different socioeconomic status or ethnic origin. The same negative attitudes may obtain toward the elderly, particularly the elderly poor.

## SOCIOECONOMIC STATUS

Socioeconomic status may well influence whether or not an individual seeks medical help. For example, Koos[9] asked families in a small town in New York if certain symptoms should be called to the attention of a physician. The 17 symptoms presented to the respondents ranged from chronic fatigue and loss of appetite to a lump in the breast and blood in the urine. The upper socioeconomic (business and professional) respondents rated almost all of the symptoms as requiring medical attention. In marked contrast, persons in the lower socioeconomic group considered most of the symptoms as not sufficiently serious to require medical care. The middle-class ratings were intermediate between these extremes.

Although some differences among social classes were expected in their attitudes toward the list of symptoms, the extent of the differences was unexpected. For example, the specific symptom of a lump in the breast was regarded as medically significant by 94 percent of the upper class, but by only 44 percent of those in the lower socioeconomic group. A lump in the abdomen was recognized as needing medical attention by 92 percent of the upper socioeconomic group as compared with 34 percent of the lower.

It is obvious from Koos' findings that many persons of lower socioeconomic status will not seek medical care when needed or will appear at the physician's office later than appropriate. In fact, Rainwater[14] has pointed out that lower-class patients seek medical care only when illness is so severe that essential daily living activities cannot be carried out. Further, they rarely seek help for psychologic problems, since these are considered inevitable and not subject to change.

Socioeconomic status may also play a major part in the disease for which the patient seeks help. Cardiovascular diseases are responsible for over one-third of the deaths in the United States among persons under 65 years of age. This disease is more prevalent among the upper class, whose affluence leads to a more sedentary way of life.[15] Here, then, is a situation in which the teaching role of the health professional can be carried out on the level of individual patient or the family unit. Cigarette smoking, psychologic stress, diet, obesity, lack of exercise, and hypertension have all been implicated as being related to coronary disease—appropriate topics for preventive health education.

Twenty-five years ago smoking was more frequent among the upper class. This situation has now reversed itself, possibly related to the fact that persons of lower socioeconomic status are less concerned or knowledgeable about research findings regarding the health hazards of smoking and may also be more interested in immediate satisfactions than remote in-time effects.

Since there is a strong relationship between social class and occupation, it will be important for the health professional to know something of his patients' work history and present working conditions. To what degree is a farmer exposed to harmful pesticides? Has the patient worked around chemicals that have been implicated in a number of diseases? Coal miners should certainly be checked for symptoms of black lung disease. Are business executives helped to handle occupational stresses that may lead to hypertension and/or peptic ulcers?


## CULTURAL DIFFERENCES

Ethnic background influences patients' attitudes toward illness and toward the professionals who care for them when they are sick. They are likely to have internalized the behavior patterns of the culture in which they matured. For example, in an interesting investigation of reactions to pain, Zborowski[22] found significant differences in the behavior of various ethnic groups. He studied patients in a large veterans' hospital in New York City. The ethnic groups in the hospital were roughly representative of those in the city. Among his findings, it was notable that the WASPs were stoical about pain and reported few emotional reactions, while patients of Jewish and Italian heritage expressed their sufferings freely and complained with little inhibition. The hospital staff tended to label the Jews and Italians as "complainers." However, Zborowski did not accept this explanation of the pain response in Jews and Italians. He found instead in his study that Italians were present-oriented, asked for immediate relief of the pain, and were satisfied when the pain was relieved. Jews, on the other hand, were future-oriented, and although they too sought relief of the pain, they were concerned about the source of the pain and its consequences for their future health.

Zborowski's work calls attention to the fact that although both Jews and Italians were regarded as "complainers" because of their emotional reaction to pain, their complaints served different functions. It was clearly demonstrated that similar reactions to pain do not necessarily indicate similar attitudes. Further, as pointed out by Mechanic,[12] the future orientation of the Jews may have positive as well as negative consequences. For example, the overprotectiveness of Jewish parents may lead to health anxiety in their children, but the same concern can also encourage high standards of child rearing.

Cultural factors may influence what the patient reports to his physician about similar diseases. Zola[24] interviewed 63 Italians and 81 Irish who were new admissions to the Medical, the Eye, and the Ear, Nose and Throat clinics before they were seen by a physician at the Massachusetts General Hospital. He found that the Italians demonstrated more diffuse reactions to being ill; they complained of more pain, reported more symptoms, and more frequently the symptoms caused them to be irritable and hard to get along with. The Irish, on the other hand, were more stoical, complained less of pain, reported fewer symptoms with greater specificity, and did not believe that their symptoms interfered with their interpersonal behavior. These differences in behavior during illness were explained by the different defense mechanisms attributed to the two cultures—the Irish using denial, and the Italians, dramatization, to cope with their problems.

Zola[23] has done further work indicating that diagnostic errors based on cultural differences may be so great as to create epidemiologic differences. The above study produced data about 29 patients (12 Italian, 11 Irish, and 6 Protestant Anglo-Saxon) in whom no organic disease could be found. Since it had earlier been determined that psychosocial problems were equally present in the three groups, there was no basis for expecting any one of them to receive a greater number of psychiatric diagnoses. However, 11 of the 12 Italian cases were diagnosed as having psychiatric problems, while a psychiatric diagnosis was attached to only 4 of the remaining 17 cases. Thus, it seems that ethnic background and the manner in which symptoms were presented influence the diagnosis. Perhaps the psychosocial problems of the Italians were overdiagnosed because of the dramatization of their symptoms. On the other hand, such problems were clearly underdiagnosed in the Irish and Anglo-Saxon groups, probably because of their stoicism. Were these latter groups possibly denied the benefits that might have resulted from referral to a mental health resource?

The Zola studies imply that the health professional needs to be aware of the influence of ethnicity when patients report symptoms, especially where diagnosis and treatment are to a large extent based on what the patient tells the physician. Important diagnostic leads might be overlooked. A patient who does little complaining about pain and describes a single symptom precisely may not appear to be in great distress.

For example, a 58-year-old woman reported pain in one knee during her routine annual physical examination. Earlier, there had been indications of mild arthritis in other joints, and the symptom was dismissed as further evidence of early arthritis, with the statement that it was "something that you'll have to learn to live with." By the time of the next annual physical examination, this woman had developed a limp and a painful hip as a result of favoring the affected knee. At this time, referral to an orthopedist was made and diagnostic studies revealed a large number of broken cartilage chips behind the kneecap. The cartilage chips were removed during the outpatient surgical procedure required for the diagnostic testing, and the pain soon subsided. However, extensive physical therapy was required to restore function to the knee and hip. Perhaps a year of unnecessary pain and the expense and inconvenience of several months of physical therapy could have been avoided had the patient been less stoical during her initial report of pain.

Zola's findings are particularly relevant for the management of chronic diseases, for which treatment is primarily concerned with control of the illness and with whatever rehabilitation may be possible. The health professional who understands that what the patient reports may be a function of ethnic background will investigate more deeply in some cases but not respond inappropriately in others. The professional will then be better able to support the patient's attempts to cope with the illness.

## MINORITY GROUPS

We have discussed under separate headings some of the ways in which socioeconomic status and cultural differences may affect health care. Here we are concerned with several of the largest minority groups in the United States. These groups carry the double burden of having readily identifiable ethnic differences and being among the poorest financially—Chicanos, black Americans, Asians, and Puerto Ricans.

## Chicanos

Clark[5] has made an extensive study of health matters among the Spanish-speaking people of San José in the Santa Clara Valley of northern California. That study resulted in certain recommendations for health professionals.

### Problems Related to Communication
It had been found that hospital staff were critical of Chicano patients who spoke Spanish among themselves. Clark recommends that they not be discouraged from doing so, since the Spanish language is a symbol of their cultural tradition.

However, health workers should not assume that all Chicanos prefer to speak Spanish. Some might take offense at the suggestion that they cannot communicate in English.

All explanatory matter should be simple and free of technical jargon. For example, a pamphlet written in Spanish explaining venereal disease control contained terms such as *"supuracion por la uretra"* (suppuration from the urethra). Such terminology is not only unfamiliar to the barrio resident, but would likely not be understood by a middle-class Anglo.

### Dealing with Folk Beliefs
Clark recommended that health workers in the barrio attempt to learn as much as possible about local medical beliefs and practices. Such knowledge would help the professional attempt to dispel those folk beliefs detrimental to health. Ridicule of folk beliefs is, of course, completely unacceptable.

At times one can work within folk beliefs. For example, mothers might not comply with a recommendation to give large amounts of boiled water to a child with diarrhea but would much more likely follow the physician's suggestion of large quantities of herbal tea, in which they have confidence.

Recommendations for sudden and marked changes in dietary habits are not recommended. Rather, different proportions of foods already being used may lead to better acceptance.

### Problems Related to Modesty
Extreme modesty is instilled in Chicano females from childhood. Consequently health professionals should avoid more exposure of the female patient's body than is necessary, and hospital beds should be screened for any examinations requiring exposure.

### Problems Related to Medical Roles
Within the Chicano culture, the individual does not make medical decisions alone. This responsibility is a family matter. Clark recommends that an older family member be included in discussions about needed medical action. Further, when a new health program is proposed, it is better to encourage the entire family or even groups of families to follow the recommendations. The individual may be more concerned about what others say than about what the health professional thinks of him.

Barrio families are more concerned about other matters than health. When a health worker is able to assist a patient in finding a job or helping a child with school problems, the patient may be more likely to cooperate in dealing with health problems.

### Problems Related to Hospitalization
Barrio people fear being hospitalized. They may not understand hospital procedures, fear isolation from family and friends, are concerned about their ability to make their needs known, and dislike the assault

on their modesty and the hospital diet. Consequently, whenever possible these people should be treated at home.

When hospitalization is necessary, they should be allowed to have family members with them as much as possible. It is helpful to put them in wards where they may communicate with other Spanish-speaking patients, although complete segregation is discouraged.

### Problems of Social Distance

Chicano patients respond best to health workers who show sincere interest in them, their friends, and their feelings. This finding suggests that the interviewing skills recommended in this book are quite appropriate for the Chicano patient. Anderson and her associates[1] support this view. Reporting on a study of the resolution of Mexican-American resistance to pediatric heart care, they state that approaches with demonstrated effectiveness in working with Chicanos include: reflection of feeling (the understanding response), a nonpatronizing use of language at the patient's level, and nonverbal skills such as good eye contact, sitting close to the patient, and nodding to indicate that the interviewer is following.

## Inner-City Blacks

Sager and associates[17] have made certain recommendations for working with black families from the inner city. Although their suggestions are not as comprehensive as those that Clark has made for Chicanos, it will be noted that there is much similarity in the two sets of recommendations.

It is pointed out that health professionals are not immune from either overt or latent racism that views the black as "different" and incapable of responsible human relationships or worthy motivation. The white practitioner's knowledge of the black family is most often based upon either secondary sources of information or minimal first-hand experience. Consequently, the white professional must learn more of the values, cultural patterns, and living conditions of inner-city blacks, preferably through increased contact. By so doing, whites may learn to understand their life-style without judging it on the basis of conventional moralistic values. For example, alcohol and drug abuse might be seen as an expression of frustration resulting from seemingly inescapable and continuing discrimination, rather than immorality.

The simple courtesies of a handshake and addressing the individual as "Mr." or "Mrs." (or "Ms.") are important signs of respect. It is inexcusably rude to address a new patient by a given name while the professional retains the title of "Doctor."

The dangers of stereotyping the behavior of black families is stressed. For example, as a generality, it may be true that an illegitimate pregnancy will cause little concern within some families; however, for a particular family the stigma may be overwhelming. Similarly, the authors of the report suggest that to assume that all black families are matriarchal is as stereotyped a view as to assume that all Jewish mothers are replicas of Mrs. Portnoy.

In the recent past, many black families preferred to consult white health professionals, considering them more competent. This situation has changed, and black families now prefer to see black professionals. The black health worker will have the advantage of a fuller understanding of the patient's culture and language. However, black practitioners will have to earn the trust of black patients just as white professionals do. They will be subject to the suspicion that now that they have achieved professional status, they may have assumed "white" values. In any case, it is not recommended that either black or white professionals treat only those of the same skin color, which in itself constitutes a racist stance. In fact, there is evidence that patients are not concerned about the race or ethnic origin of their physicians, provided competent care is provided. In one study,[2] interviews were conducted with 66 patients (40 black, 21 white, 5 Mexican-Americans) of three family physicians (Asian, black, white) at a clinic providing care to low-income and welfare patients. No differences in patient satisfaction were found among the three racial groups, regardless of which physician had been seen. Patients did agree that they appreciated their physicians' competence, caring, listening, and understanding of what they had to say. They did not believe that these qualities were a function of the physician's race.

Thomas[20] makes the interesting observation that a black person's survival in the United States may depend on the development of a "healthy" cultural paranoia. Similarly, hostility has served as a coping mechanism. Consequently, when confronted with suspiciousness or hostility in a black patient, one should recognize that this behavior may not be directed so much at the health professional as at the stereotype of the white person. In general, Thomas finds that the interviewing skills discussed in this text are most appropriate for use with black patients. Further, for successful work with black families, the major effort should be the avoidance of behavior and attitudes indicative of racism, rather than changes in skills or methods of practice.

## Asians

In Chinese, Japanese, and Korean families there is much emphasis on certain duties and obligations. When these traditional expectations are violated (eg, disobedience to parents and other authority, low achievement, divorce, occurrence of psychopathology), shame befalls the family.[4] The extreme guilt and ensuing depression in those who have caused this disgrace is frequently masked by minor somatic complaints. When these persons come for medical care, they are likely to emphasize the bodily symptoms rather than the guilt and depression.[10] In his work with East Asian patients, Tseng[21] has found that to concentrate on the depression arouses so much guilt that the problem is exacerbated. However, if the somatic complaints are accepted and treated, the depression may show a spontaneous remission, or the patient may be more willing to deal with the psychologic problem.

With their background of obedience to authority, Asians come to believe that to be a "good" patient, one should not complain of pain or demonstrate anger; they should be grateful for the care they receive. Consequently, all health professionals who deal with Asians may have to anticipate their feelings ("That must hurt very much"; "You must be annoyed with me for being late"), rather than wait for overt expression of these feelings. Similarly, since hospitalized Asians are not likely to buzz for the nurse, nurses may have to look voluntarily into the rooms of these patients more often to evaluate their needs.[4]

Chang[4] points out that, with Asian patients, it is most important to avoid the use of closed questions that can be answered with a "yes" or "no." "Yes" is apt to mean that the patient is listening, but not necessarily understanding. The use of negative questions should especially be avoided. The example is given of a nurse asking, "Haven't you gone to x-ray?" A "yes" answer from an Asian patient may mean "Yes, you are right, I haven't gone to x-ray."

## Puerto Ricans

Physicians and nurses will need to be aware of the hot-cold theory of disease in dealing with Puerto Rican and other patients from the Carribbean. Belief in this theory has also been observed in some Mexican-American communities. If an illness is classified as "cold," it is treated with "hot" medicines and foods, and vice versa. A study of Puerto Rican patients carried out by the Martin Luther King, Jr. Neighborhood Health Center in the South Bronx demonstrated that these patients simply will not take their medications on an outpatient basis if their prescription or recommended food or liquid violates this theory.[13] Similarly, Harwood[8] has shown that noncompliance in following a prescribed drug regimen is very high when these beliefs are not understood by the physician.

Fortunately, some standard medical care accommodates easily to the hot-cold theory, since the patient's beliefs coincide with the treatment that would ordinarily be recommended. A Puerto Rican ulcer patient will readily accept a bland diet because ulcers (a "hot" disease) would not be treated with "hot" spicy foods. On a similar basis, aspirin (a "hot" medication) would be acceptable for colds and arthritis ("cold" diseases).[8]

When standard treatment differs with the hot-cold theory, accommodation is frequently possible. For example, the "hot" effect of penicillin can be neutralized by recommending that it be taken with cool liquids.[6] Since a cold should be treated with "hot" remedies, hot tea or soup can be prescribed rather than the usual "plenty of fruit juices" as a means of forcing fluids.[13]

## DANGERS OF STEREOTYPING

The previous discussion of socioeconomic and ethnic characteristics implies that some aspects of the behavior of each individual will resemble that of other members of that person's group. Although partially true, such an assumption can lead to stereotyping. It is quite likely that there will be as great variations within groups as between groups. The presence or absence of an ethnic speech accent, the patient's education and occupation, and the number of generations since immigration to this country may provide the health professional with clues about the extent to which the patient shares group values and attitudes.

The import of our discussion of socioeconomic and ethnic differences is this: the physician or nurse is likely to understand and to react more favorably to the tractable, conforming, middle-class patient than to the "difficult" patient of different status. However, since the professional's responsibility to the "difficult" patient is the same as to the cooperative patient, an understanding—and acceptance—of differences is essential. Lock[10] suggests that, since health professionals cannot be experts in medical and cultural sociology and anthropology, they must make every effort to understand the meaning of the illness to the patient, regardless of the patient's ethnic or class background. She cites the case of a first-generation Greek immigrant who is the mother of a 20-month-old obese child. Although this mother believes her baby to be healthy, during each visit to her pediatrician she is encouraged to change the child's diet to bring about a weight reduction. She cannot accept this recommendation. She believes that a fat baby is the model of good health and maternal care, and a demonstration of her family's prosperity. Consequently, she is seeking a new pediatrician. If the mother's belief system had been explored and accepted, and if the pediatrician had explained the reasons for weight reduction to her, a more favorable outcome might have been effected.

## WORKING WITH THE ELDERLY

"No community can call itself civilized if it treats its older generation with a lack of consideration. But consideration requires understanding, and everyone needs to know more about the process of aging and the difficulties it may bring."[18]

This quotation from a 1981 report on aging in Great Britain would hardly raise one voice of dissent. Yet, in spite of general agreement, there is evidence of widespread misunderstanding and subtle prejudice against the elderly. These attitudes, which determine, to a large extent, the kind of treatment older individuals receive, have come to be known as "ageism."[11] "Ageism" can lead to the kind of stereotyping discussed above: people over 65 are considered slower, duller, and more frequently ill, dependent, helpless, and hopeless than other groups. Clearly, while this description may be true of some, it is certainly not true of all and, unless perceived as an illogical judgment, can do harm by discouraging individual assessment. Nor is it a secret that some professionals have "ageist" attitudes and find caring for old people less rewarding than working with younger patients. They therefore take less time for careful diagnosis and treatment, attributing some symptoms, which in younger people would merit considerable study, to "You're just getting older."

These factors led us to place this commentary on the care of the elderly, who are actually as diverse a population as any, with that on the groups discussed earlier. The elderly, too, can experience avoidance and "distancing" by professionals.

Fortunately, certain developments are forcing increased attention to the elderly and their needs. The population statistics, in themselves receiving more and more publicity, are one factor furthering better care. At present, the elderly (over 65) constitute about 11 percent of our country's population. By the first third of the next century, they will reach the 25-percent mark. Significantly, their numbers are increasing more rapidly than those of any other segment in the population.[7] Another—and telling—way of presenting the statistics compares certain current figures with those from the past, say 1900. In that year, a woman's life expectancy was 48, a man's, 46. In 1984, the figures are 77.1 and 69.3 years, respectively. In 1900, 3.1 million Americans were over 65. Now, 24.5 million have achieved that age. By the year 2000, the number is expected to be nearly 32 million.[16]

This impressive increase in longevity is in itself a tribute to general advances in medicine, which have benefited the entire population. At the same time, gerontology, although not yet a separate medical specialty, has established programs in medicine and other disciplines (psychology, sociology, social work) in response to the increased numbers of elderly requiring care. It is estimated that over 80 percent of older Americans suffer from at least one chronic disease, and many have two or more.[3] In time, the very need and the pressure of numbers will dictate expansion and improvement of services.

In the meantime, for many of the elderly, particularly the poor, a longer life has not necessarily meant a better life. As health and the ability to care for oneself decline, dependency increases. The first and most immediate source of help is, of course, the family. Contrary to occasional media reports of relatives' indifference or negligence, the evidence is that a high percentage of families do care and give care to their elderly as long as they possibly can.[11] It is reported that, although 20 percent of the elderly spend some time in nursing homes (often for a period of recuperation following surgery or fracture), only 5 percent of the population are actually long-term residents in institutions. However, 5 percent represents 1.4 million people, a not insignificant number.[7] And, as Dr. Robert N. Butler, former director of the National Institute on Aging, states: "The remaining 4.2 million, although living in the community, are most at risk of needing institutionalization. A change in family-support arrangements, a disabling accident, a worsening of circulatory problems or mental capacity, or other changes in ability to manage on one's own may be the precipitating cause of institutionalization" (p. 183).[3]

The nursing home, now used as a last resort for the care of the most seriously disabled, is likely to become, in the future, the haven for a considerably larger population. These facilities present a wide range in size, service, and quality. Suffice it to say that the horror stories of mistreatment of the helpless aged, housed and fed in substandard conditions, while not entirely in the past, are now rare exceptions. Present-day facilities, regulated and subsidized by federal and state governments, tend to be humane providers of basic care. Some also offer additional services, such as recreational programs, physical therapy, and social services. Yet, as Butler[3] explains, these institutions, still in an early stage of development, are similar to acute-care hospitals in the nineteenth century. The leap forward in acute care began with the collaboration between hospitals and medical schools. Humane care developed hand in hand with competence and research. If nursing homes enter into a similar association with medical schools, similar results can be expected. The diseases and deterioration of old age can be studied as quality care develops.

The needs of the elderly in institutions are not essentially different from the needs of those still living in the community, even though independence is no longer possible. Physical needs are more easily identified: competent, considerate medical care, a clean and comfortable environment, adequate nourishment, reliable and prompt help with necessary daily living activities. Psychologic and social needs are less obvious, although equally important. The elderly require continued contact with family and friends, participation in appropriate activities, and availability of counseling and those services that nourish and maintain self-respect. To meet these needs, an integrated network of services inside the facility and outside in the community are necessary.

Professionals who choose to work in the field of gerontology will use the same interpersonal skills as their colleagues who serve younger people. They will need, perhaps, an added measure of patience in dealing with slower responses. Since the field of gerontology, somewhat more than other specialties, requires an interdisciplinary approach, the gerontologist's training and practice will require not only knowledge of the other disciplines, but also of appropriate collaborative work.

## SUMMARY

Health professionals are likely to establish a relationship of openness and responsible participation with patients of similar socioeconomic and ethnic status. With those of different status, however, they may respond with less attention and concern because of inability to understand and accept their values and life-styles.

Many persons of lower socioeconomic status will not seek medical care when needed, or will consult a professional later than appropriate. Socioeconomic status may also play a major part in the disease for which the patient seeks help, since certain illnesses are more prevalent among each of the socioeconomic groups.

Ethnic background may influence patients' attitudes toward illness and toward the professionals who care for them when they are sick. However, similar reactions during illness do not necessarily indicate similar attitudes.

The professional who understands that what the patient reports may be a function of ethnic background will avoid diagnostic errors by investigating more deeply in some cases, but not by responding inappropriately in others.

Suggestions are made for working with specific minority groups—

Chicanos, black Americans, Asians, and Puerto Ricans. The major concern should be avoidance of behavior and attitudes indicative of racism rather than changes in skills or methods of practice.

It is quite likely that there will be as large variations in attitudes and behavior within socioeconomic and ethnic groups as between groups. Consequently, to avoid stereotyping, the health professional should determine to what extent each patient shares group values and attitudes.

Physicians and nurses should attempt to familiarize themselves with the various groups in their communities from which their patients are likely to come and be honest in perceiving and managing their own attitudes toward difference.

The elderly are included in this commentary on minorities because they, too, may experience avoidance and distancing in their contacts with professionals. As the group increasing most rapidly in the population, their very numbers are furthering greater attention to their needs. While most aged persons are cared for by their families and other resources in the community, more and more are expected to need long-term care in nursing homes. Therefore, these facilities will require improved and expanded programs using a multidisciplinary approach.

## REFERENCES

1. Anderson BG, Toledo JR, Hazan N: An approach to the resolution of Mexican-American resistance to diagnostic and remedial pediatric heart care. In Chrisman NJ, Maretzki TW (eds): Clinically Applied Anthropology. Boston, Reidel Publishing Co, 1982
2. Bertakis KD: Does race have an influence on patients' feelings toward physicians? J Fam Pract 13:383, 1981
3. Butler RN: The teaching nursing home: a new concept. In Bernstein E (ed): Medical and Health Annual. Chicago, Encyclopaedia Britannica, 1983
4. Chang B: Asian-American patient care. In Henderson G, Primeaux M (eds): Transcultural Health Care. Menlo Park, Addison-Wesley, 1981
5. Clark M: Health in the Mexican American Culture. Berkeley and Los Angeles, Univ of Calif Press, 1970
6. Currier RL: The hot-cold syndrome and symbolic balance in Mexican and Spanish American folk medicine. In Martinez RA (ed): Hispanic Culture and Health Care: fact, fiction, folklore. St. Louis, Mosby, 1978
7. Fromer MJ: Why docs stay away. New Physician, 11, April, 1984
8. Harwood A: A hot-cold theory of disease: implications for treatment of Puerto Rican patients. JAMA 216:1153, 1971

9. Koos EL: The Health of Regionville. New York, Hafner, 1967
10. Lock M: The relationship between culture and health or illness. In Christie-Seely J (ed): Working with the Family in Primary Care. New York, Praeger, 1984
11. McDonald DE, Christie-Seely J: Working with the elderly and their families. In Christie-Seely J (ed): Working with the Family in Primary Care. New York, Praeger, 1984
12. Mechanic D: Response factors in illness behavior. In Millon T (ed): Medical Behavioral Science. Philadelphia, Saunders, 1975
13. Murillo-Rohde I: Hispanic American patient care. In Henderson G, Primeaux M (eds): Transcultural Health Care. Menlo Park, Addison-Wesley, 1981
14. Rainwater L: The lower class: health, illness, and medical institutions. In Millon T (ed): Medical Behavioral Science. Philadelphia, Saunders, 1975
15. Rakel RE: Principles of Family Medicine. Philadelphia, Saunders, 1977
16. Reichel W: Care of the elderly. In Taylor RB (ed): Family Medicine: Principles and Practice, 2nd ed. New York, Springer-Verlag, 1983
17. Sager CJ, Brayboy TL, Waxenberg BR: Black Ghetto Family in Therapy. New York, Grove Press, 1970
18. Secretary of State: Growing Older. London, Queen's Printer, 1981
19. Simmons O: Implications of social class for public health. In Jaco EG (ed): Patients, Physicians and Illness. Glencoe, Ill, The Free Press, 1958
20. Thomas DN: Black American patient care. In Henderson G, Primeaux M (eds): Transcultural Medical Care. Menlo Park, Addison-Wesley, 1981
21. Tseng WS: The nature of somatic complaints among psychiatric patients: the Chinese case. Compar Psychiatry 16:237, 1975
22. Zborowski M: People in Pain. San Francisco, Jossey-Bass, 1969
23. Zola IK: Problems of communications, diagnosis, and patient care: the interplay of patient, physician, and clinic organization. J Med Educ 38:829, 1963
24. Zola IK: Culture and symptoms: an analysis of patients' presenting complaints. In Millon T (ed): Medical Behavioral Science, Philadelphia, Saunders, 1975, Chap 47

# chapter 12

# Death and Dying

Theoretically the interviewing skills discussed in earlier chapters should be appropriate and sufficient for communicating with the dying patient. An understanding approach is as necessary for the terminal patient as for any other. Death and dying are as much a part of medical practice as birth and living. Then why do we include a special chapter on communication with and psychosocial management of the dying patient? Simply, our experience with medical and nursing students indicates that they can master the skills of acceptance and understanding with most patients, but when given the task of interviewing a patient with a terminal diagnosis, they "freeze," become confused, leave the patient's bedside at the earliest opportunity, and experience great difficulty in reporting their interviews. Furthermore, most physicians and nurses in practice do no better.

Our impotence in the face of the inevitability of death naturally arouses our deepest anxieties and explains what otherwise seems irrational and inhumane behavior. The poet Dylan Thomas[59] wrote, "Do not go gentle into that good night. Rage, rage against the dying of the light" (p. 128). His powerful statement captures the universal sense of outrage at our helplessness.

Our behavior toward death and the dying, albeit unintentional, often is characterized by depersonalization, denial, and avoidance. These attitudes can derive only from extreme anxiety, confusion, and fear. Several factors seem significant in explaining such reactions. One is the well-known cult of youth and vigor. Their opposites—age and disability—are inevitably repugnant, and we long to escape both. Escapism works no better in this circumstance than in others and deprives us of the balm of psychologic preparation through facing and examining our fears and repugnance. A more accepting perspective might allow us the grace of a greater humanity toward those who are dying and more equanimity toward our own inevitable end.

# ATTITUDES TOWARD DEATH AND DYING

## Denial of Death

> *Doctor, doctor, will I die?*
> *Yes, my child, and so will I.*

The candid acceptance of death in this old nursery jingle contrasts sharply with prevailing attitudes toward dying. In fact, our present society has been labeled a "death-denying" one.

We have learned that death is a topic to be avoided in conversation and, when it is discussed at all, we tend to use euphemisms such as "passed away" or "expired." Funeral homes use cosmetics on the dead to make them appear to be sleeping, and the bodies are shown to visitors in "slumber rooms." Newspapers have reported that there are, unbelievably, drive-in funeral homes where the body may be viewed and the guest book signed from one's car—a further commentary on a society that attempts to deny death by making it as distant and as mechanical as possible.

Hospitals may institute elaborate measures to disguise the fact that a patient has died. When the hospital loudspeaker or visual call system announces a death in code, nurses station themselves at elevators and stairways to control the flow of traffic, permitting the hasty removal of the body to the morgue without detection.

A time study has shown that nurses take twice as long to answer the buzzer of a dying patient as compared to a call from one with a more favorable prognosis. Perhaps the most extreme form of denial is the cryogenic movement, whose motto is "Freeze, Wait, Reanimate." Members of this group believe that death is completely unnecessary. Corpses are placed in liquid nitrogen to await discovery of cures for the diseases that caused the deaths. It is assumed that by that time science also will have discovered how to restore life to a frozen body.[15]

## Misconceptions About Death and Dying

Weisman[63] has compiled a list of ten generally prevalent attitudes toward death and dying, based upon interviews with medical practitioners in various specialties:

  1. Even when death is inevitable, no one is willing to die, unless he is suicidal or psychotic.

2. Since reconciliation with the necessity of death and preparation for death are impossible, one cannot help another to accept death.
3. Fear of death and dying is the most natural and fundamental fear. The closer one comes to death, the more intense the fear becomes.
4. Talking of death with the dying removes hope and may hasten his demise.
5. If asked about death by a terminal patient, a physician should turn questions aside and use any means to deny, rationalize, and avoid open confrontations.
6. The fact that dying patients do not ask about their prognosis means that they do not want to know about it. Unwelcome disclosure may involve the risk of suicide, psychosis, profound depression, or severe regression.
7. When recovery is impossible the patient should be left alone, except for relief of pain. In this manner, he will gradually withdraw from the world and die in peace.
8. A physician's scientific training, clinical experience, and knowledge of pathology enable him to deal with all aspects of terminal care, including the emotional and psychological.
9. If the family does not wish a patient to be told his diagnosis and prognosis, the physician should abide by that decision. Psychological problems can be effectively managed with simple reassurance, adequate sedation and, when death is imminent, referral to the clergy.
10. After the patient dies, the family is no longer the responsibility of the hospital or physician.

Weisman labels these attitudes as "misconceptions, or at least unwarranted generalizations." The remainder of the discussion in this chapter will attempt to document that, in general, they are indeed misconceptions.


## Current Changes in Attitudes Toward Death and Dying

There are indications that the attitudes just discussed are changing. One sees television programs and articles in popular magazines and newspapers on this formerly taboo topic with increasing frequency. During the past 15 years more articles on death and dying have been published in professional journals than during the previous hundred years. Three centers have been established in the United States to promote scientific and humanistic inquiries, as well as the dissemination of knowledge of the psychosocial aspects of dying, reactions to death, loss and grief, and recovery from bereavement. There are two journals—*The Journal of Thanatology* and *Omega*—devoted exclusively to the problems of death and dying.[15]

Courses relating to death are now offered in high schools and colleges.[28] An Iowa journalist, noting the insensitivity of friends to his own cancer condition, founded an organization called Make Today Count, in which groups of terminally ill patients meet regularly for mutual support, lectures, etc.[29] In Berkeley, California, a hotline has been established, manned by 100 volunteers, many of whom are terminal patients themselves. This service provides 3500 hours of free counseling per month to the dying and their families.[64]

Kübler-Ross and Nighswonger[33] report increased interest and cooperation in their research on the dying over a period of several years. When they first approached the staff of a large teaching hospital for permission to interview terminal patients for their studies, they were informed that there was not a single dying patient in the hospital! At the start of their research it took many hours of effort to get permission to interview a terminal patient. Within three-and-one-half years this time was reduced to less than an hour. Currently they receive referrals from physicians, nurses, social workers, and patients who have themselves experienced the value of expressing their feelings about impending death. Here then is evidence that in the context of a hospital where teaching seminars are conducted, a climate of openness can be developed, permitting the staff to modify their own fears and guilt.

In summary, it may be stated that attitudes are changing slowly from viewing death as a subject to be denied and hidden to a willingness to face it with honesty and an interest in compassionate inquiry.

## PSYCHOSOCIAL MANAGEMENT OF THE DYING PATIENT AND THE PATIENT'S FAMILY

Terminal care refers to the management of patients for whom the imminence of death is believed to be certain and for whom no further medical effort is considered effective. In a positive sense it becomes concerned with the patient's comfort through relief of pain and other symptoms and the emotional support of both patient and family. When practiced negatively, terminal care starts when the physician says that nothing more can be done and begins to withdraw from the patient.

Broadly stated the aims of terminal care are, for patients, to assure that they die with as much peace of mind, dignity, and freedom from suffering as the disease process permits; for the family, to provide necessary support so they feel that everything possible is being done, to involve them in such a way as to prevent later guilt that they may not have played their proper part, and to protect them as much as possible from unnecessary hazards of bereavement.

Management of the dying patient in these terms gives full meaning to the concept of comprehensive medicine. Such care will require health professionals to take an interest in the relevant social, emotional, economic, and religious aspects of a patient's life. Terminal care, more than any other problem of health management, will require maintenance of a relationship based on confidence and trust, permitting the dying patient to express feelings and thoughts freely. Health professionals will need to demonstrate honesty and understanding, while remaining composed and calm.[17]

Specific aspects of the psychosocial management of the terminally ill will be discussed below: prolonging life and permitting death; talking with the dying about death; the stages of dying; working with the family of a dying person; aftermath of bereavement; working with the family during bereavement; and facilities for the psychosocial management of the dying.

## Prolonging Life and Permitting Death

### Death with Dignity

If we accept the premise that death with dignity is one of the major goals of terminal care, then we must ask candidly if extraordinary methods or "medical heroics" should be used to prolong life for, at best, a brief period. Death with dignity implies that all ordinary means should be used to preserve life, even when there is no reasonable hope for recovery, but that extraordinary means need not be used when cure is impossible and suffering is prolonged. This principle implies that life is a fundamental good, but that life that may be no more than painful breathing should not be perpetuated beyond all other considerations. In other words, the duty to preserve life is relative, not absolute.

The late Pope Pius XII stated that there is no obligation for the physician to go beyond usual means of treatment. The Church Assembly Board for Social Responsibility avers that it breaks no unalterable Christian law if, on the principle of loving his neighbor as himself, a physician allows a person to die.[25]

### Rationalizations for Use of "Medical Heroics"

Kübler-Ross[32] wonders if the desperate attempts by health professionals to deny impending death by the frequent concentration on machines and equipment is based upon the fact that "machines . . . are less close to us than the suffering face of another human being, which would remind us once more of our lack of omnipotence, our own limitations and fallibility, and, last but not least perhaps, our own mortality?" (p. 8).

Baltzell[1] describes a newborn infant, a genetic monster, kept alive following a tracheotomy and gastrostomy performed a few days after birth. This "child" lingered in the special care unit of the nursery until death, months after birth. The young parents were not only left deeply in debt, but their own suffering was prolonged as they watched painful but ineffective procedures administered to their child.

Similar events occur regularly—continual diagnostic testing despite the clear inevitability of death, daily blood tests to confirm what is already known, chemotherapy for terminal cancer patients, and heroic cardiac procedures.

It is the repeated observation of measures such as these that has led health professionals themselves to question their usefulness. For example, Quint[47] observes: "When you see . . . relatives suffering prolonged agony watching a member of their family go downhill, stay downhill, financially unable to afford care, emotionally drained, you realize that death can be a blessing—not only to the person who is the patient but to those who love him" (p. 167). In the same vein Shepard[57] states: "A rational, compassionate person cannot witness the human suffering and indignity that occurs in institutions that provide long-term care without questioning the ethics supporting the prevention of death and the prolonging of a life that has become hopelessly wretched" (p. 22).

The unwillingness to terminate heroic procedures frequently is rationalized on the basis of not wishing to "play God." The same author asks, "Is not the use of a monitor on an 83-year-old man in congestive heart failure a kind of espionage in a battle with the Almighty?" (p. 25). Baltzell[1] is more emphatic when he states, "The physician who initiates the chain of events leading to the intensive care unit must assume more responsibility for initiating the decision as to when to turn off the machines. The cruel travesty of the moribund patient kept alive yet denied sufficient narcotics to ease his pain because his death might thus be hastened should cease" (p. 107).

### The Dilemma of Defining "Extraordinary Means"

The advances in medical science and technology have led to ethical dilemmas for the health professional. The Reverend Paul B. McCleave,[37] former director of the American Medical Association's Department of Medicine and Religion, clearly points out the physician's dilemma:

. . .there is the paradox of the patient who has been in an oxygen tent, has been in a coma from seven to eight weeks, has received blood, liquids for nourishment, tubes for elimination. His body is burning up with fever, and he is being eaten away by cancer. That which was a body of 125 pounds is now down to 82 pounds. Why? Is this life? What is life? Isn't there any dignity in death? Don't I have a right to die? Doctor, when I'm in that position, don't continue with such measures, because I have a right to die in dignity. What is the problem in our professions—are we afraid of death? Is this why we continue to prolong life, because we are afraid? As doctors, we need to recognize that just because someone dies, we are not failures. I am sorry, Mr. Physician, but the Creator at the very beginning of time decided that we were going to die and there is nothing we can do about it—each man dies. I'm not advocating mercy killing, or euthanasia. I'm talking about permitting a person to have the dignity of death without suffering and pain. I know that the church has said, "Well, Doctor, don't worry. You don't need to use extraordinary measures, just use ordinary things to maintain life." But the strange part of it is, what was extraordinary yesterday is ordinary today and what is extraordinary today is going to be ordinary tomorrow in medical practice (p. 2).

In an attempt to resolve the above dilemma, Reich[52] suggests that the following factors should be considered in deciding whether an effort might be considered extraordinary: (1) A reasonable hope of success. (2) The strain, pain, and discomfort accompanying a given treatment or procedure, recognizing that these reactions may vary from patient to patient. (3) The need for consciousness in one's terminal condition, which might include the patient's justifiable wish to go home and "die in peace" with the family. Denial of this request would constitute an extraordinary means of preserving life. (4) The cost of the procedure. (5) External factors, such as preservation of life to assure just inheritance. (6) Special reasons of conscience, such as religious convictions that prohibit blood transfusions. Reich himself recognizes that these guidelines are not infallible. He offers them in an attempt to "create attitudes that are favorable to the right to die with dignity which, after all, is not very different from the right to live with dignity" (p. 39).

Thus, in the absence of infallible guidelines, the physician's own wisdom and clinical judgment, not the family's guilt, misinformation, or unwarranted hope, become the determining factors in the decision to abstain from further intervention. Recently, however, it has been recognized in some areas that this responsibility ought to be shared and physicians have therefore been provided opportunities to review these decisions with other professionals. For example, an Optimum Care Committee for helplessly ill patients has been established at Massachusetts General Hospital.[46] Beth Israel Hospital in Boston has established carefully spelled-out principles for "orders not to resuscitate."[48]

### Withholding Consent for Heroics

Just as one may withhold consent, while conscious, for surgery, blood transfusions, and other medical procedures, Margaret Mead[38] suggested making a legal statement, while one is of sound mind, withholding consent for ". . . medical intervention which may result in states which, while called life, nevertheless mean a life without meaning" (p. 20).

A professor of medicine[58] has executed such a statement. He quotes from a letter he wrote to his personal physician many years ago:

> If I become ill and unable to manage my own affairs, I want you to be responsible for my care. To make matters as simple as possible, I will leave certain specific instructions with you.
>
> In the event of unconsciousness from an automobile accident, I do not wish to remain in a hospital for longer than two weeks without full recovery of my mental faculties. While I realize that recovery might still be possible, the risk of living without recovery is still greater. At home, I want only one practical nurse. I do not wish to be tube-fed or given intravenous fluids at home.
>
> In the event of a cerebral accident, other than a subarachnoid hemorrhage, I want no treatment of any kind until it is clear that I will be able to think effectively. This means no stomach tube and no intravenous fluids.
>
> In the event of a subarachnoid hemorrhage, use your own judgment in the acute stage. If there is considerable brain damage, send me home with one practical nurse.
>
> If, in spite of the above care, I become mentally incapacitated and have remained in good physical condition, I do not want money spent on private care. I prefer to be institutionalized, preferably in a state hospital.
>
> If any other things happen, this will serve as a guide to my own thinking.
>
> Go ahead with an autopsy with as little worry to Ev as

## Directive to Physicians

Directive made this _____ day of _____ (month, year).

I, _____ being of sound mind, willfully and voluntarily make known my desire that my life shall not be artificially prolonged under the circumstances set forth below, and do hereby declare that:

**(a)** If at any time I should have an incurable injury, disease, or illness certified to be a terminal condition by two physicians, and where the application of life-sustaining procedures would serve only to artificially prolong the moment of my death and where my physician determines that my death is imminent whether or not life-sustaining procedures are utilized, I direct that such procedures be withheld or withdrawn, and that I be permitted to die naturally.

**(b)** In the absence of my ability to give directions regarding the use of such life-sustaining procedures, it is my intention that this directive shall be honored by my family and physician(s) as the final expression of my legal right to refuse medical or surgical treatment and I accept the consequences from such refusal.

**(c)** If I have been diagnosed as pregnant and that diagnosis is known to my physician, this directive shall have no force of effect during the course of my pregnancy.

**(d)** I understand the full import of this directive and I am emotionally and mentally competent to make this directive.

Signed _____

Social Security Number or Birthdate _____

Street Address _____

City, County, and State of Residence _____

### *Witness*

This directive must be signed by two witnesses. The following persons *may not* serve as witnesses: **(a)** anyone related to the declarer by blood or marriage, **(b)** anyone entitled to a part of the declarer's estate, by will or otherwise, **(c)** anyone with a claim against the declarer's estate, **(d)** the declarer's attending physician, or any of the physician's employees, **(e)** the employee of a health facility (hospital or nursing home) in which the declarer is a patient.

\*\*\*\*\*

The declarer has been personally known to me and I believe him or her to be of sound mind.

Witness _____

Witness _____

Witness _____

Witness _____

This directive complies with the Natural Death Act, chapter 112, Washington Laws of 1979. However, additional specific directions may be included by the declarer.

**Figure 1.** The "living will" developed as part of the natural death act of the State of Washington *(From Geyman JP: Dying and death of a family member. J Fam Pract 17: 125, 1983.)*

possible. The Anatomy crematory seems a good final solution
(p. 54).

Although this physician's statement indicates his wishes clearly,
he could at that time have no assurance that his doctor would comply.
With the passage of the Natural Death Act in 1976 in California, such
"living wills" were legalized. According to California law, a physician
who does not agree with a patient's instructions to stop "heroic" treatment must withdraw from the case and turn it over to another physician.[18] Other states have since followed California's lead.

In Figure 1, we reproduce the "living will" developed as part of the
Natural Death Act of the State of Washington, enacted in 1979.[17]

## Talking of Death with the Dying

### Basic Assumptions

We base our discussion of what to tell terminal patients about their
illness on the following assumptions: (1) The patient has the responsibility for decisions about managing his or her life. By depriving him or
her information about prognosis, the physician denies the patient the
opportunity for informed choice among possible alternatives. (2) One's
body is certainly as much one's property as one's home or car. Although
the facts about the body are determined by health professionals, the
body still belongs to the patient. (3) The physician–patient relationship
should be based on mutual respect and confidence. If information is
withheld from the patient, the ethical basis of the relationship is violated. (4) A terminally ill patient has certain responsibilities to discharge before death—making peace with God, settling personal affairs, as well as making provision for the family. Fulfilling these
responsibilities will be denied a patient who does not have information
about his or her terminal condition.[45]

If these assumptions are accepted, it should follow that providing
information in an appropriate manner would also be a recognized part
of the physician's obligation to the terminally ill. However, research
findings indicate that most physicians believe patients should not be
told of their terminal prognosis. Oken[40] found that 90 percent of physicians preferred not to tell their patients, primarily because of emotion-
laden a priori judgments. The information given also varies with the
kind of illness. Evasion is employed with 75 percent of cancer patients
but with only 25 percent of heart patients.[11]

## Do Patients Wish to Know?

By contrast, other findings reveal that the majority of patients feel they should be told. In one study reported by Kelly and Friesen,[30] three distinct groups were interviewed at a cancer detection center. Of 100 cancer patients all of whom knew their diagnoses, 89 percent were pleased they had been told; 6 percent would have preferred not to know; 5 percent had no opinion. Of 100 noncancer patients, 82 percent would want to know the truth if they had the disease and 14 percent would not. Among a group of 740 patients undergoing diagnostic tests at the cancer detection center, 98.5 percent wanted to be told the truth.

This disparity between what patients want and what physicians do is significant. Physicians' motives are not in question, only their underlying attitudes toward death and what these dictate as far as practice is concerned. An interesting sidelight on physicians' attitudes toward revealing fatal prognoses is that a majority feel that they themselves would like to be given complete and honest information under similar circumstances. Their rationale is that as physicians they possess greater emotional stamina as well as greater responsibilities than the average person. However, physicians are no more frank when their fellow physicians are terminal patients.[25]

## Rationalizations for Withholding the Truth

It is frequently stated that the truth should be kept from the patient in order to prevent possible suicide. Hinton[25] argues that the fear of suicide is exaggerated:

> If frank discussion were often to result in patients becoming severely or persistently distressed, even suicidal, few doctors would wish to speak with them of dying. There does tend to be an exaggerated fear that dying patients will kill themselves if they are told their illness may be fatal. The chances are that the suicidal acts which occur in those with mortal disease are due to the suffering and the spiritual isolation when the sick are lonely, rather than any despair following a sympathetic discussion of their outlook. Although suicide remains a threatening possibility, inhibiting some from frank discussion with the dying, it is hard to find a case where a humane conversation on these lines precipitated any suicidal act. It is much more likely to have prevented it. "I know what I'd got," said a young woman who had attempted suicide, "I'd seen it in my notes. I'd looked it up in the medical books and knew I couldn't recover. I wanted to talk about it with the doctor, but he

always seemed too busy, or just called it inflammation" (pp. 137–138).

Hinton's comment that it is hard to find a case where humane disclosure of the truth precipitated suicide is supported by Litin's study[35] of all the suicides during a 10-year period at the Mayo Clinic. Although only one case of suicide appeared related to a patient being told he had cancer, thousands of patients had been told of the same diagnosis during this 10-year period.

Nurses frequently state that they avoid discussion of death with a terminal patient because they cannot violate the physician's order not to reveal diagnoses. However, as Benoliel[5] suggests: ". . . talking with a person to clarify what he thinks is happening or to understand his worries is not equivalent to telling him his diagnosis; rather it is the one way to learn what is on his mind" (p. 266). Even if the patient should ask directly, "Am I going to die?" the nurse (or any other health professional) need not retreat. The patient, in all probability, is seeking an opportunity to express fears and concerns, rather than wanting only a direct answer (see discussion of The Trap of the Question Mark, Chapter 3).

There is strong evidence that patients who know of their terminal conditions derive real benefit from this knowledge. In an effort to evaluate the effects of telling patients that they have a terminal illness, Gerle and associates[16] told one group of patients that they had inoperable cancer while another group was not told. An impressive majority (87 percent) of those who were told was able to maintain emotional balance, as judged by a psychiatrist. Some in this group were upset initially but soon regained their composure. In both groups there were equally small numbers of patients who never achieved serenity. None of the patients in the group that was told reacted in an excessive manner. The social worker, who continued to visit the patients and their families throughout the illness, reported improved family relationships among the group that had been told. There was also less tension and desperation with the progressive deterioration than in the group that was uninformed.

### Patients "Know" More Than They Are Told
Many patients come to know of their terminal conditions even when they do not ask and are not told. Hinton[24] interviewed 102 patients on a weekly basis during their terminal illness and found that on his first visit nearly half knew what was happening. This awareness grew so that 75 percent eventually spoke of the possibility or certainty of

dying. None of these patients had been told by a professional and the ward staff were frequently unaware that they had this knowledge.

Saunders[53] has stated, "The doctor who believes that patients only 'know' what he tells them is deluding himself" (p. 386). Patients know their prognoses not only from direct words but also from what is happening in their own bodies and from the attitudes of health professionals and family—their silences, their efforts at false reassurance, evasions, and denials.

Dying patients will ask no questions, however, when they know that they will not get answers but only reassurance that communicates to them that the health worker is either unable or unwilling to talk about dying. For example, Hackett and Weisman[21] studied 20 patients dying of cancer who had not been told of their terminal condition. Yet all 20 revealed during psychotherapy that they knew they were dying. When questioned as to why they had kept silent about it, the typical response was that they assumed the physician and family members did not wish to talk about it. It almost seems that these patients joined in the conspiracy of silence to protect the physician and family from their discomfort.

Since patients come to an awareness of their own dying whether they are explicitly told or not, they will tend to lose confidence in health professionals who withhold information. Patients must then tolerate their fear with little or no emotional support and without the therapeutic effects of open and honest communication.

### Consequences of Differing States of Awareness

Glaser and Strauss[19] have described four different states of awareness: *closed awareness,* in which the patient does not yet recognize impending death, although others do; *suspected awareness,* in which the patient suspects what others know for certain; *mutual pretense awareness,* in which both the patient and others know that death is imminent but behave as if they did not; and *open awareness,* in which all parties, including the patient, know the truth. In each of these contexts the quality of relationship between patient and hospital staff is different.

When awareness is closed there is a conspiracy of silence and avoidance among hospital personnel, physician, and family members. The patient's environment is controlled by duplicity, social games, and contrivance. If the patient discovers, traumatically or inadvertently, that he or she has been deceived and is, in fact, going to die, there may be an explosive transition to awareness that disrupts professional and family relationships. Both the patient's panic and the staff's anxiety may then need to be managed by the busy physician. As Hinton[24] has suggested, prevarication and empty reassurance stimulate distrust and loneliness.

In the context of suspected awareness the patient is engaged continually in a contest for information with the hospital staff. Staff members attempt to control their contacts with the patient so that information is not given inadvertently. Distance is maintained and relationships are impersonal. Questions are met with evasion, vagueness, expressionless features, and the inevitable, "Ask your doctor." Hospital personnel are prevented from being sincere in their relationships with patients by these implicit or explicit rules against providing information.

Mutual-pretense awareness provides a modicum of dignity and privacy for the dying patient. The staff are relieved of some of their more elaborate deceptions and their anxiety may be reduced. However, the patient must bear the burden of tact and discretion in not admitting the foreknowledge of death. This situation obviously benefits the staff rather than the patient. No one can long sustain such a social game or cater to the convenience of others by his or her manner of dying.

Related to both suspected awareness and mutual pretense awareness is "middle knowledge." The patient indicates by speech—inconsistencies, contradictions, and slips of the tongue—that indeed, he does have some knowledge of what is happening in spite of the conspiracy of silence of his caretakers. In the words of Hackett and Weisman,[22] "He is between knowing what his body tells him means death and what those around him deny is death" (p. 303).

The state of open awareness has advantages for both patients and hospital staff. There are implicit standards of conduct; staff have to be accepting and professional, and under these conditions patients can manage to abide by certain rules for their way of living while dying. In one research setting[14] the patients all knew they were going to die and their deaths were an open and everyday topic of conversation. These patients were able to provide mutual support for one another, to receive support from the hospital staff, and even to support the staff when *their* anxieties were aroused.

Open awareness is preferred even by children. Vernick and Karon[62] describe a program on a leukemia ward at the National Cancer Institute in which every child over the age of nine was told the diagnosis as soon as it had been verified. The children accepted the information, sometimes with obvious relief. They were thereafter free to express further concerns and all questions were honestly answered. All

51 children in the program functioned well. Withdrawal and depression occurred infrequently and was usually transient.

Physicians and nurses must accept their own human limitations. Some of their patients are going to die. Health professionals cannot avoid their own anxiety in any way that will be constructive for their patients. Therefore physicians and nurses need to be aware of their own reactions to dying and death and give careful thought to the way their feelings affect their patients.

## Initiating Discussion

The beginning of communication about anticipated death should be started early. Prior to surgery or other major treatment, the physician can indicate how critical the illness is. The patient is thereby given the option to inquire about the threat involved and the possible efficacy of treatment.

The physician who wishes to disclose a fatal prognosis to the patient must not be abrupt. Aware of the fact that most patients almost certainly have considered death as a possible outcome, the physician might remark, "I suppose you've been wondering how ill you really are." Should the patient deny concern, the physician might continue with, "Well, perhaps we should look at it together." Such a comment usually will elicit from the patient a statement somewhat like, "You mean it's that bad?" However, if a patient indicates a wish not to consider it, that wish should be respected. The physician has indicated his willingness to be open and frank, and the patient is free to raise the matter when he or she feels up to it. In either case the patient has been permitted to come to the truth at his or her own rate. The health professional should also be sensitive to a patient's somewhat ambiguous comments that indicate readiness to discuss a terminal prognosis. For example, a man might state that he has heard a good deal about donating one's body to science or to a medical school or that his portfolio of stocks and bonds will provide adequately for his wife. If the health worker responds in an open-ended manner, eg, "Is there some reason why you are interested in that at this time?" the patient may take the initiative if he wishes to continue. In this manner, the interviewer can determine how much the patient knows or wishes to know.[10] Once the possibility of frank discussion has been provided, the patient will feel sufficiently secure to give the health professional the needed clues. Since the pace and the content of the clues will vary from patient to patient, the approach of the health worker must be individualized, not routinized.

Once patients know that their illness is fatal, they need time to assimilate what this means for them. Both patients and family members will have many questions to ask and many feelings to express. Each of their concerns needs to be dealt with patiently and often repeatedly. The physician, who cannot always be available for extended handling of such feelings, can alert the nurse and tell the patient that the nurse will be available during the physician's absences. Such collaboration relieves the nurse's doubts about what the physician expects. Further, it provides for a shared responsibility between physician and nurse with obvious advantages for both. More important, however, is the consistent care it offers the patient.

Because uncertainty is difficult to tolerate, one of the questions patients and family frequently ask is a precise estimate of survival time. However, until reliable criteria for such prognoses have been established, estimates of life expectancy should be given with extreme caution. Parkes[42] found that prediction of survival time was unrelated to the actual length of survival. Further, 83 percent of the "errors" were in the optimistic direction, the patient being expected to live longer than actually was the case. These optimistic predictions may have represented a wish to reassure patients and relatives and, by extending expectations unrealistically, to provide new hope.

### Reaction to Dying as a Function of Age

The elderly frequently show increased personal acceptance of death as a natural process, and some may even welcome death as an appropriate end to a full life or to prolonged suffering. Young patients who are dying demonstrate different, although age-appropriate, emotional reactions. When health professionals understand and anticipate these reactions of the young, they will be better equipped to help them in their struggles with the fact of dying.[12]

Children below the age of six generally have no clear concept of the reality of death. They perceive death as a reversible process. Their life experiences tend to confirm this concept of reversibility. A television "bad guy" may be shot dead in today's program only to reappear on the next. Pets that have died often are replaced immediately. Because of their naive belief in the reversibility of death, preschool children approach personal death with relative serenity. The greatest support will have to be given the parents rather than the child.

The grade-school child generally perceives death as a separation but still a continuation of physical existence. Since children may have been told that a deceased parent or other close adult is "happy in heaven with God," they are likely to react with a sense of abandonment. If the child then becomes fatally ill, the role of the health professional is to deal with the anxiety and fear of separation from loved ones.

The teenager understands the meaning of death but finds it intolerable to accept personal death. A teenager may be in acute conflict over the need to turn to others for comfort just as beginning independence is emerging. The health worker should be prepared to help the adolescent with this additional conflict between dependency and self-sufficiency.

Rage is the most typical reaction to impending death for young adults. After having completed preparation and training for what lies ahead, they naturally look forward to what they will be able to accomplish and enjoy. "They are so ready to live that to them death is a brutal, personal attack, an unforgivable insult, a totally unacceptable solution to any illness or any treatment procedure" (p. 204).[12] The task of helping fatally ill persons in this age group to achieve some acceptance may well prove the most demanding for the professional.

The essential, underlying principles of open and honest discussion of dying do not vary from age group to age group. They must be applied flexibly, however, with due regard to differences in the meaning of death at the various stages of life. Each case requires reorientation of the professional, if the patient is to make the transition from a focus on death to a renewed perception of the life that still remains.

## The Stages of Dying

Kübler-Ross[32] has found that dying patients go through sequential but overlapping stages. Awareness of these stages and the behavior and feelings likely to appear at each of them will assist the health professional in providing the appropriate support and understanding that may enable the patient to achieve a state of relatively peaceful acceptance.[39]

### *Denial*
When first conscious of a terminal illness, although perhaps years away from death, patients typically go through a state of shock and denial. They behave as if they did not hear what they cannot accept emotionally. The "No, it can't be me" response to news of a terminal diagnosis may be a self-protective reaction to shock, permitting a patient time to gain sufficient strength to cope with an overwhelming situation. The patient should be permitted this initial denial, which may last from a few minutes to months. However, prolonged denial can be fostered by health professionals who, for their own comfort, reinforce the patient's need to pretend that the diagnosis is not true. If the stage of denial is unduly extended, the patient may avoid further treat-

ment, since treatment is not necessary for a condition that does not exist. Panic is the alternate response to denial. The patient demonstrates impulsive and unrealistic behavior and may see no way out except through psychosis or suicide. These reactions usually result when the patient has been abruptly told of the terminal diagnosis and the informer does not remain available to absorb the initial shock.

### Anger

If denial is not reinforced, patients eventually find that it cannot be sustained. As they perceive progressive deterioration in their physical condition and functioning, denial is replaced with anger. The patient displaces anger freely with no apparent reason. Physicians may be told they have mismanaged the treatment, nurses and visitors are told that they do not come often enough or that they disturb the patient who is trying to rest, there are complaints about the quality and frequency of meals, and God has forsaken the patient too. The "No, it can't be me" changes to "Why me?" Unfortunately, external controls are frequently placed on the verbal expression of anger as though it were a dangerous acting-out. Patients are met with evaluative responses in which they are told of the inappropriateness of this behavior, while God and the dietary staff are defended. Visitors and nurses resort to counterhostility by threatening not to come at all. The outcome of such reactions is that patients turn the anger inward resulting in depression and accompanying feelings of guilt and unworthiness. However, health professionals who recognize that the patient's behavior is *displaced* anger will be in a position to accept and encourage its expression as appropriate for one in the patient's plight. Similarly, the patient's family should be made aware that anger directed toward them may also be displaced. The family members then may be less likely to respond in kind, thus facilitating progress toward the next stage.

### Bargaining

When the anger is permitted free expression it soon abates, and patients enter the stage of bargaining in which they try to negotiate a "deal" with God, with the physician, or with the nurse. Perhaps God will change the course of the disease process itself. Or, perhaps, if the patient is highly cooperative, the staff will make extra efforts, or a new treatment will be discovered that will result in a cure. Sometimes the negotiation is to postpone death until a certain purpose has been achieved (completion of a will or a toy being made for a child) or a certain event has taken place (a daughter's wedding or the patient's own birthday). Such patients have now moved to the "Maybe not me" stage. For patients whose anger was suppressed in the previous stage, the depression that follows results in "selling out" rather than in bargaining. They come to believe that they are receiving what they deserve, or depressive withdrawal becomes so intense that they assume a "What's the use?" attitude. For the patient who is trying to negotiate a bargain, it is important not to reinforce this unrealistic effort by giving false hope. Rather the health professional should remain a sensitive and understanding listener as the patient struggles with attempts to postpone the inevitable. The bargaining stage is usually characterized by calmness and comfort for the patient.

### Depression and Preparatory Grief

The stage of bargaining is a relatively short one. The progress of the illness serves to remind patients that they are indeed dying. As they begin to accept the reality of what is happening, they enter the stage of depression and preparatory grief. Having acknowledged impending death, "It *is* I," a patient must go through the process of mourning for him- or herself. At this point the health worker may be tempted to resort to inappropriate reassurance: "Don't cry, it's not that bad." But it *is* bad to leave everyone and everything one has cherished. Just as it was useful to permit and encourage the expression of anger in the second stage, it will now be helpful to permit and encourage crying and the expression of grief. When the sadness is characterized by silence, sitting quietly and holding the patient's hand will provide assurance that the patient has not been abandoned while coming to terms with the inevitable.

### Acceptance

Patients who have not been helped through these normal stages (for example, the patient who "sold out" in the third stage), will by now have resigned themselves to a meaningless end to existence. In contrast, the patient who has successfully completed the first four stages will enter the stage of acceptance, now free to live while dying rather than die while living.

Krant[31] has stated that in order to die with dignity

> people need to feel in control of their lives during the dying time, to feel dignified enough to participate in decision-making and feel esteemed enough to interact supportively with their family and friends. In return, the environment must be supportive to allow meaningful interchange to occur (p. 27).

These conditions appear to be present in the circumstances of a woman who had already lost the use of one leg from a cancerous growth that was spreading. Her story, presented by her physician for publication,[4] is entitled, "How to Exit Laughing." The following is an excerpt.

My doctor looked down at his hands for several moments and then, when he did look up at me, said soberly but gently, "Well . . . move, if it will relieve your mind in any way . . . but I wouldn't sign a lease."

The lease would have been for a year, so I was being told I had perhaps a year, certainly not much more, to live. I appreciated the warning. If you were going to Europe or anywhere far away to stay a long while, wouldn't you want to get things in order, make all the arrangements and plans? Of course, I'm having a great time here and really hate to leave, but perhaps I have overstayed a bit, judging from the daily obituaries. I am on my way to 70 and, as the Marine captain said when they were taking Okinawa (legend has it), "Come on; what'sa matta with youse guys, you wanna live forever?"

My four brothers and four sisters have long since departed, which means I can no longer relive our childhood days without being a mouthy bore. I begin to notice there is no one around who remembers anything any more, and when my young neighbor asked me the other day, "Who is Greta Garbo?" I felt it was indeed time to get ready.

. . . I have felt well enough at times to have guests in for cocktails and sometimes some of the family for dinner. I love to cook and I love to play bridge, and it is a joy to be able to do both. What if I cannot play golf (my husband says that distorts the picture, because I never could) or garden an acre, or go on good 2-mile bird-watching binges the way I used to? I'm alive and having a wonderful time . . . .

While the deliciousness of living is highlighted because the party is almost over, I have all these good days to get ready to go. I can go through and sort some of my books and reread some of them . . . I can sort out all my jewelry and leave a piece in an envelope for special friends.

. . . No awkward intruder will invade my privacy posthumously because I am lucky to have gotten the word. I can stand a while yet on my good-byes . . . in a word, I have the rare opportunity to look around again and see how wonderful it all is and then, actually, to see myself off. What more could anyone ask? (pp. 1040–1042)

## Working With the Family of a Dying Member

Family members may go through the same stages as the dying member. Therefore health professionals should be available to the family so that their attitudes do not negatively affect the patient's progress through the various stages of dying. For example, a family fixated at the stage of anger may prevent or delay the patient's eventual acceptance. Consequently, it will be in the interest of both family members and patient if they can be helped to experience the various stages at approximately the same rate.

All family members should know the truth about the patient's terminal condition. Frequently health workers tell only the spouse, assuming that he or she will adequately inform children and others. Since the spouse may be under severe stress, other members of the family either may not be informed or be told in a manner that produces unnecessary anguish.[49] When the terminal condition of the patient is quite certain, it may be an appropriate time for a family conference, providing the physician with an opportunity to observe which of the family members requires special help.

Family members should also be involved and kept informed of decisions about treatment. This procedure will be useful in preventing unnecessary guilt feelings following the death.

Working with the family should usually be the responsibility of the primary-care physician. It is assumed that this physician will have had a continuing relationship with the patient as well as the other family members, and will be in a better position to "take charge" than one or another consultant who may have been called in to see the patient but has not known the family. It goes without saying that family members who wish to talk directly with the consultant should have the opportunity to do so, provided the primary-care physician continues in the described role.

## Aftermath of Bereavement

### Normal Mourning
Just as there are stages of dying, so are there stages of mourning. Brown and Stoudemire[7] note that the three stages of mourning follow a predictable course. The first stage, *shock,* helps to shield the bereaved from experiencing the loss too quickly or too intensely. This stage may last from a day to several weeks. The bereaved feels dazed, helpless, and disorganized. The shock is probably more intense in the case of a sudden or unexpected death.

The emotional numbness of the first stage gives way to fully experiencing the loss. This ushers in the second stage, *preoccupation with the deceased.* Each phase of the past relationship is carefully recalled and examined—pleasure, grievances, anger, neglect, guilt. Social isolation is also typical. The second stage usually becomes apparent about three weeks after the death and may last for up to six months. Symptoms of this stage may reappear on anniversaries of the death.

The third stage, *resolution,* is characterized by cheerful recalling of past events involving the deceased. An increasing interest in activities in the present usually begins. Social contacts are resumed and somatic symptoms (loss of appetite, weakness, fatigue, insomnia) decrease.

### Pathologic Mourning

An awareness of the stages of the grief process will enable the health professional to note if bereavement is progressing normally or if signs of pathology are being indicated by delayed or distorted mourning. *Delayed mourning* can be manifested either by an absence of overt grief or a belated onset, suggesting that feelings are so intense that they are being repressed or denied. Survivors are frequently reinforced in this behavior by friends and relatives who comment on how well they are "bearing up." Those who experience delayed grief frequently are later subject to acute feelings of loss on the anniversary of the death. These individuals tend to develop symptoms of a major depression while denying that they are grieving.

*Distorted mourning* may be manifested by one or more of the following: (a) prolonged mourning, which may last for years or even a lifetime, (b) lack of communication of feelings of grief within the family, (c) failure to resume usual work, school, or social activities, (d) identification with the dead person to the extent of acquiring symptoms associated with the last illness of the deceased, (e) continued preoccupation with the deceased (frequent grave visits, leaving the room of the deceased "as it was"), (f) deterioration of physical health, (g) inability to speak or hear of the dead person without crying even a year or more after the death, (h) severe depression.[7, 34, 36]

Pathologic mourning is frequently seen in obsessive personalities who have difficulty in expressing emotion. Survivors whose relationship with the deceased was marked by ambivalence or hostility may feel great guilt, viewing the death as a fulfillment of their "death wishes."[7] The driver in an automobile accident in which his bride was killed, even though he was not at fault, blames himself for her death. Excessive guilt in such situations puts the bereaved at greater risk for pathologic grief.

### Morbidity and Mortality among the Bereaved

There is now reliable evidence that the bereaved are more vulnerable to morbidity and mortality in the year immediately after loss. This evidence provides health professionals with valuable opportunities for crisis intervention and preventive medicine.

Parkes[41] has reported that the incidence of widows seeking consultation with general practitioners for psychiatric symptoms tripled in the first six months after bereavement; the rate for nonpsychiatric symptoms increased by half.

A more serious outcome of bereavement is the probability of early death of survivors. Rees and Lutkins[51] studied the death rates in a single community in Great Britain for a six-year period. Mortality among bereaved close relatives (spouse, child, parent, or sibling) was compared with a control group matched for age, sex, and marital status. It was found that close relatives died within one year of bereavement seven times more frequently than in the control group. The increase in mortality was particularly great for widows. During the first year of bereavement, 12.2 percent of widows died compared with 1.2 percent in the control group. (Perhaps Sir Henry Wotton[65] observed the same phenomenon when he wrote:

> He first deceas'd; she for a little tri'd,
> To live without him; lik'd it not, and di'd.)

A more recent study in Washington County, Maryland, showed similar findings. Helsing and Syklo[23] prospectively studied 4032 widowed persons and a like number of married persons, matched for age, sex, race, and place of residence. Widowed men in all age groups experienced higher mortality rates than the married men. The differences reached statistical significance in the age groups between 55 and 74.

In Great Britain, a study of 4486 widowers[43] suggests that many literally die of a "broken heart." In the first six months of bereavement, their death rate was 40 percent higher than the expected rate for married men of the same age. Fully two thirds of the increase in mortality was found to have resulted from heart and circulatory disorders that developed after the death of the spouse.

The connection between the death of one spouse and the sickness and death of the surviving spouse has long been recognized. The physiologic basis of this connection has only recently been demonstrated. A group of researchers at the Mount Sinai School of Medicine[56] conducted a prospective study on 15 men whose wives were dying of breast cancer. They found a significant decline in the activity of lymphocytes (white blood cells involved in the body's disease-fighting system) during the two months after the death. Thus, the immune function of the widowers was lower than before the wives' deaths, even though the husbands had known that their wives' cancer was terminal. A year after the deaths, lymphocyte responses had not returned to their former levels. It is not clear how bereavement affects lymphocyte function. The stress of grief or changes in nutrition, exercise, sleep, and drug use are suspected causes.

## Working with the Family During Bereavement

As the person most immediately available to the bereaved at the time of the death, the role of the health professional during the shock stage of mourning is to encourage and accept the first expressions of grief. Crying can be therapeutic and should receive an empathic response. As the family members begin to think of practical steps that must be taken, they should be helped to participate in funeral arrangements. Many physicians feel that they have given adequate attention to the bereaved when they have prescribed a sedative. Although mild sedation may be advisable, an overuse of drugs can mask or delay grief, thus prolonging the process of mourning.

Help with completing the second stage of mourning (preoccupation with the deceased) is best carried out by other family members and friends. However, if the bereaved is alone, or if the family network blocks the expression of grief, the health professional should encourage regular visits during this period of stress.[7] The concerned health worker can, during these meetings, facilitate the expression of grief and thus prevent it from becoming an unresolved source of mental or physical anguish. Shakespeare gives poetic and poignant expression to the need for verbalizing grief: "Give sorrow words: the grief that does not speak knits up the o'erwrought heart and bids it break" (Macbeth, Act IV, Scene 3).

Recognizing the morbidity and maladjustment following bereavement, Raphael[50] studied the effectiveness of preventive intervention. She gave support to the expression of sadness, anger, hopelessness, helplessness, and despair. The mourning process was facilitated by reviewing the positive and negative aspects of the lost relationship. Raphael's study showed a significant lowering of morbidity in the intervention group compared to the control group. In a similar study, Cameron and Brings[8] demonstrated that those who received bereavement counseling showed significantly fewer emotional signs of distress and less counterproductive coping strategies than controls. Self-help support groups (in which participants help each other find ways of living with widowhood) are known to be effective, as are confidant groups (which facilitate the development of close friendships between pairs of widows).[2]

When one of a couple dies, the surviving spouse should be encouraged whenever possible to share living arrangements. Payne[44] points out that the suicide rate of surviving spouses living alone is three times greater than that of persons in the same age group who are not bereaved.

Special care should be given to children in the family. Children should not be told that the dead family member "has gone to sleep for a long time." Children who associate death with sleep may become phobic about going to bed. In a similar fashion, children who are told that a sibling or parent was taken by God are apt to identify God with loss.[9] Children above the age of five or six should share in the family grieving and be allowed to attend the funeral of a parent or sibling. When the truth is kept from children, they may imagine something considerably worse than the reality, even to the point of feeling some personal responsibility for the death.

Engel[13] offers useful practical suggestions as to how the empathic nurse may work with the bereaved. He suggests that news of the death is best communicated to a family group rather than to a single individual. The disclosure should take place in privacy where the family members may react without the constraints of public display. The nurse who feels unable to handle this task because of unresolved feelings about death should attempt to enlist the aid of another professional.

If the family members wish to see and take leave of the dead person, the request should not be denied on the basis that it may be too upsetting. This request will not be made by those who will find it unbearably disturbing.

When berated by angry relatives who accuse the nurse, the physician, or the hospital of mismanagement, the professional should avoid becoming defensive. These complaints are likely to represent guilt and possibly hostility toward the dead person. Recognizing that the accusations of the relatives are not directed against him or her as a person, the nurse will be able to demonstrate necessary tolerance and understanding.

Knowing that shock and disbelief may be the initial response to the death, the nurse may anticipate that some family members will behave in a disturbed manner. The nurse's patient, gentle restatement of the reality and a demonstrated wish to help will assist the bereaved with the difficult task of acknowledging the truth of the situation.

Ideally, working with the bereaved should begin before the patient dies. The greater the opportunity to express feelings prior to the actual death, the more bearable it becomes later. Through such anticipatory mourning, especially in extended illnesses, the grief process may be almost complete before the death.

## Facilities for the Care of the Terminally Ill

### Hospital Care

With the development of aggressive therapeutic attitudes and the emphasis on active use of beds, especially in teaching hospitals, terminal care has come to be regarded as a misuse of hospital facilities. "There is nothing to be learned from a patient for whom nothing more can be done," is a frequently heard comment. These attitudes are understandable in light of the following factors: (1) Too many deaths on an acute ward disturb the other patients. (2) The presence of the slowly, but obviously, dying has a similar effect. (3) Deaths cause heavy and unpleasant physical work for nurses, who are often under pressure because of other responsibilities. (4) The terminal patient is not happy on an acute ward. The tempo is wrong, with no one available for the important tasks of listening and understanding.

In some hospitals dying patients are isolated within a ward by removing them to a side room. This procedure has the advantage of simplifying medical and nursing care, but it only increases the patient's isolation. Further, the transfer to such a room is not lost on other patients and can have a generally depressing effect.

As a consequence of the unwillingness of most hospitals to become involved in terminal care, more of the elderly are relegated to nursing homes. However, these homes may not be any better prepared to handle dying patients than the acute hospital (see Working with the Elderly, Chapter 11).

### A Small Specialized Hospital

A small specialized hospital for terminal care has several advantages: (1) The staff can become experts in terminal management. (2) Since there is no reason for a curative role, staff can concentrate on symptomatic treatment and psychosocial care. (3) Concentration of groups of similar cases would facilitate research. (4) It could remove much strain from hospitals for acute illnesses.

One of the authors (L.B.) had the opportunity several years ago to visit such a small, specialized hospital, regarded as a pioneering institution in the development of terminal care procedures. St. Christopher's Hospice in Sydenham, South London, England, is a 54-bed terminal-care facility that treats families as units and cares for the surviving members during bereavement.

Space will not permit detailed description of the cheerful, optimistic environment generated by the tasteful architecture, the gardens, the congenial staffing arrangements, the nondenominational chapel, etc. Of greater import is the immediate impression that this is one of the most cheerful hospitals one has ever visited. The atmosphere is more alive and friendly than in hospitals where patients are far less desperately ill. The practice at St. Christopher's on admission is to make the patient feel welcome from the moment of arrival. The patient is greeted at the door by name by the matron. A warmed bed rather than a cold, impersonal stretcher or cart has been prepared and has been wheeled to the entrance as the patient arrives. Such procedures may be the first steps in demonstrating to patients that they matter and that they are going to be respected as persons.

Control of pain is emphasized. Analgesics are given regularly rather than on demand, based upon a schedule that prevents pain from occurring rather than controlling it once it is present. In other words, drugs are given to relieve pain for a period slightly longer than the chosen routine time. Even when diamorphine is given prophylactically to prevent the return of otherwise intractable pain, it is very unusual to encounter true psychologic addiction. Patients do not develop a craving for the drug when they no longer are desperate for relief from their pain. Consequently drugs are never prescribed on a pro re nata basis.[60]

Sherry is served to patients before the afternoon and evening meals and alcohol has an important place in treatment. The medical director of the Hospice has stated, "It [alcohol] is often the best sedative for the elderly and should also be employed for the opportunities it gives for social exchange. Man is a social being and will still find gratification in being convivial or in a relaxed moment with family or friends" (p. 168).[54]

With symptoms controlled and pain not permitted to recur, patients regain an interest in life and turn to those personal activities that are meaningful for them. Relatives, including young children, are welcomed at any time, and they may be taken into the gardens to enjoy the open air, the flowers, and the fish pond. Here one can see patients and their families interacting comfortably with the children of the Playgroup, whose mothers work in the Hospice while they are competently cared for. It becomes obvious that the patients are not set apart and that the wall behind which the dying are so frequently "hidden" does not exist here.

It is important that patients establish close bonds with one or more caretakers. However, it cannot be known in advance to which staff members a patient will relate best. Therefore, every person on the staff is viewed as important, including the aides and volunteers. The usual formal relationships among hospital staff are absent. Much attention is paid to the special needs of patients. For example, Goldin[20] reports that a patient at St. Christopher's whose trachea had been eroded by disease was given enormous gratification in his final days by being offered as often as he wished ice cubes flavored with a variety of tasty substances including, best of all, whiskey! Religious tolerance is shown by the fact that patients are free to use bedside earphones to listen to regular radio programs if they wish to "tune out" ward prayers. In spite of such individualized services, the cost of maintaining a bed at St. Christoper's is 50 to 60 percent of the cost of a bed in a teaching hospital (St. Christopher's operates an active teaching program for medical, nursing, and theological students) and 60 to 70 percent of a general hospital bed in the same area.[55]

Most terminal patients wish to die at home, but families are understandably fearful of undertaking this responsibility. At St. Christopher's, every possible help is given to families in caring for the dying patient at home, whenever circumstances permit. The development of a family service support team has meant that as many patients can receive the services of the Hospice at home as in the hospital. Visits at home by members of the health care team are assured, as is readmission whenever necessary. To permit patients to remain at home as long as possible, a day clinic has been established for the management of pain, physiotherapy, and socialization.[20]

Interviews with patients confirmed that their pain was so well controlled that it did not recur. Yet none of the patients appeared oversedated. They were alert and occupied with personal interests, individually or in groups. All patients interviewed called attention to the marked contrast between their present care and manner of living to that experienced earlier in large hospitals.

One could not leave this cheerful, friendly place, where no patients were oversedated or attached to machines or had tubes inserted in them, without feeling that there was much to be said for emphasizing the *quality,* rather than the *length* of life that remained for these terminal patients. Geyman[17] has characterized this kind of care as "careative" rather than "curative."

### A Special Unit within a Hospital

Goldin[20] points out that hospices will never be able to meet the huge need for humanistic care of all dying patients. She feels that hospitals must eventually provide similar care, with hospices assuming the role of teaching.

In New York City, St. Luke's Hospital has established a multidisciplinary team that attends dying patients in their regular hospital beds. A hospital in London is carrying out a study to determine whether a separate ward for the dying is preferable to the New York St. Luke's model.[20] In both instances, care is centered in the hospital. This solution may have the merit of demonstrating the concerned care given to patients by the hospice teams within the hospital. The demonstration might serve to teach and motivate the entire hospital staff to be equally caring of *all* patients.

### The Hospice Movement in the United States
Although the hospice movement began in Great Britain, where there are now approximately 70 hospices in operation, the enthusiasm has spread to at least five continents.[20] There are over 1000 hospices operating in the United States at the present time. American hospices differ from the British in that most of them do not have inpatient facilities. Rather, they exist as teams of physicians, nurses, clergy, psychiatrists, social workers, and volunteers who provide medical care as well as emotional support to families caring for patients at home, and are usually available on a 24-hour-a-day basis.

From another point of view, dying at home with hospice help is less costly than dying in a hospital. For almost 500 home patients attended by the New Haven Hospice, the average total cost of services for the last three months of illness was less than the cost of a week's stay in the hospital. Inpatient hospice care is about 27 percent less than in acute hospitals. The cost factor has not gone unnoticed by the federal government; in 1983, hospice care was approved for Medicare patients, in an effort to control the constantly rising costs of that program.

### Evaluation of Hospice Care
Hinton[26] compared patients dying of Hodgkin's disease and leukemias in three different facilities in London, each chosen for its good reputation, but differing in communication policies. Patients at one facility, a hospice, could readily discuss their condition and the probability of dying. At the Foundation Home for cancer patients, there was greater reticence about discussing cancer or dying unless patients were clearly intent on knowing. At the third facility, the radiotherapy wards of an acute hospital, frank talk about dying was infrequent. It was found that patients were less depressed and anxious at the hospice, and preferred the more frank communication available there.

Vande Creek[61] analyzed the first year of operation of the home-care hospice of Columbus, Ohio. It was found that over 90 percent of patients were satisfied with each of the items examined: care and supportiveness of the nurses; the social worker's helpfulness; symptom control (primarily pain); contribution of volunteers. Further, it was found that the cost was competitive with that of skilled nursing-home care.

Although patients generally evaluated the home-based Fairview Hospice in Minneapolis favorably, 40 percent reported difficulty in relating to or getting information from their physicians. This finding suggests that, as with any treatment, hospice care will be successful to the extent that the staff believes in and carries out its concepts.

## *Home Care*

It is generally agreed that, other things being equal, the terminally ill should be cared for and die at home. Terminal care at home can be quite adequate if the following suggested criteria are met: (1) Physicians must be satisfied that home care is appropriate and that they can cope with the medical aspects. Home care will usually mean that there has been a prior period of assessment or treatment in the hospital. (2) There must be full agreement of the patient and the family, who must understand the amount of work and anxiety they will have to face. (3) Supporting services must be available, eg, visiting nurse, hospice team. In applying these criteria, the possibility of intermittent hospital readmissions should be considered, not only for reassessing means of controlling symptoms, but also to provide relief to a hard-pressed family.

Until about 1900, most Americans died at home, permitting family and children gradually to face the fact that death would come. Children took over tasks for the dying patient. After death, the body remained at home for several days so that friends and relatives could visit. Allowing death to be a family event, the sick member drew comfort from the support of the family, and the pain of bereavement was eased by the recollection that the support had been fully and freely given. These observations may explain the finding that the death rate of close relatives within a year after bereavement is significantly reduced when the death occurs at home.[51]

Many sociologic factors are making terminal care at home less and less frequent.[15] Progress in medical science and extension of health services has increased the number of elderly persons. While the number of elderly is increasing, their place of residence is less and less likely to be with children or grandchildren. The extended family (several generations living together) has been replaced by the nuclear family (parents and children). Consequently, the death of an elderly person is less likely to take place at home under these modern family conditions. Since deaths occur primarily among the aged, the former accepted custom of dying at home has changed to dying in health care institutions. At the present time, approximately 80 percent of deaths occur in hospitals or nursing homes.[17] The number of persons dying in institutions may be expected to grow larger in view of increased medical benefits for the aged and the continued segregation of the elderly from their families.

In discussing deaths within nuclear families, Holland[27] cites studies indicating that advanced cancer patients have a strong need for closeness and affection from spouse and other family members, and suggests that the terminally ill be kept at home as much as possible. He further recommends the development of hotel-like facilities near hospitals, which would permit the patient to live with the family and go to the hospital clinics for necessary treatment.

To compare costs of hospital and home care, Bloom and Kissick[6] compared a sample of 19 patients who died at home and matched them with patients who died in a hospital. For the two weeks preceding death, hospital costs were 10.5 times greater than those of home care. This difference was in large part based upon the greater range and larger quantity of diagnostic and therapeutic procedures provided hospital patients until the day of death. Cost did not appear to be the motivating factor for those who selected home care; both groups of patients were covered by Medicare or Blue Cross.

Perhaps the import of the above discussion is that adequate psychosocial management of the terminal patient is not so much a function of locale or type of administrative arrangement as it is the conviction of those caring for patients that death and dying can give opportunity for rewarding professional work; they are not simply the end products of failure.

## SUMMARY

Students and professionals in the health sciences can master with comparative ease the skills of acceptance and understanding with most patients. However, when confronted with a terminal patient they experience great difficulties in communication and in providing adequate psychosocial management.

The behavior of health professionals toward the dying is often characterized by depersonalized, inhumane denial and avoidance. This behavior is a reflection of prevailing attitudes of our society, which has been described as a "death-denying" one. There are indications that within the past several years attitudes have begun to change slowly toward a willingness to face the subject of death and dying with honesty and an interest in compassionate inquiry.

*Terminal care* refers to the management of patients for whom the imminence of death is believed to be certain and for whom no further medical effort is considered effective. Concern centers on the patient's comfort through relief of pain and other symptoms and on the emotional support of both patient and family.

Death with dignity implies that all ordinary means should be used to preserve life, even if there is no reasonable hope for recovery, but that extraordinary means need not be used when cure is impossible and suffering prolonged. The very advances in medical science and technology themselves have led to the ethical dilemma of how to define what constitutes "extraordinary means," since what is extraordinary today may be ordinary tomorrow. Although guidelines for resolving this dilemma have been suggested, they are perforce relative rather than absolute. In the absence of infallible guidelines, physicians must use their own wisdom and clinical judgment in the decision to abstain from further intervention. Fortunately, hospitals are beginning to establish multidisciplinary committees to assist in these difficult decisions. Further, legal or quasilegal documents have been developed in which the patient may, before becoming terminally ill, request to have "medical heroics" withheld.

Providing information about prognosis in an appropriate manner should be an accepted part of the health professional's responsibility to the terminal patient. Yet there exists the peculiar paradox that a significant majority of physicians believe patients should not be told of their terminal prognoses, while an equally significant majority of patients wish to know the truth. There is no evidence to support the rationalization that the truth should be withheld because of the risk of suicide. On the contrary, there is direct evidence that patients who have been told compassionately of their terminal conditions are benefited. Different degrees of patient awareness will affect the quality of the relationship with health workers.

The beginnings of communication about anticipated death should be started early. Revelation should not be abrupt, and the approach must be individualized rather than routinized. Physician and nurse can share this responsibility. Open and honest discussion of dying will permit the patient to make a transition from a focus on death to a renewed perception of the life that still remains.

Awareness of the normal stages of dying and the behavior and feelings likely to appear at each of them will assist the health professional in providing appropriate support and understanding to enable the patient to achieve a state of relatively peaceful acceptance. In this manner a death with dignity may be achieved, especially if communication is maintained with the patient's family.

The responsibility of health personnel should not be considered completed on the death of the patient. Grieving relatives will need to express their feelings of loss and hurt, anxiety, depression, anger, and guilt, just as the patient has. There is now reliable evidence that the bereaved are more prone to morbidity and mortality in the year or two immediately after loss. This evidence provides health professionals valuable opportunities for crisis intervention and preventive medicine.

Although dying should preferably occur at home, a series of related sociologic factors—the increase in the number of elderly persons whose place of residence is less likely to be with children or grandchildren and the majority of deaths occurring among the aged and not, as in the past, among younger elements in the population—is making terminal care in institutions more prevalent. Fortunately, the hospice as an institution for the care of the terminally ill is attracting much interest. Adequate psychosocial management of the terminal patient is not primarily a function of locale or type of administrative arrangement. More important is the conviction of those caring for the patient that death and dying can provide opportunity for rewarding professional work.

# REFERENCES

1. Baltzell WH: The dying patient: when the focus must be changed. Arch Intern Med 127:106, 1971
2. Barrett CJ: Effectiveness of widows' groups in facilitating change. J Consult Clin Psychol 46:20, 1978
3. Barzelai LP: Evaluation of a home based hospice. J Fam Pract 12:241, 1981
4. Bean WB, Featherman K: A time for dying. Current Med Digest 37:1039, 1970
5. Benoliel JQ: Talking to patients about death. Nursing Forum 9:255, 1970
6. Bloom BS, Kissick PD: Home and hospital cost of terminal illness. Med Care 18:560, 1980
7. Brown JT, Stoudemire GA: Normal and pathological grief. JAMA 250:378, 1983
8. Cameron J, Brings B: Bereavement outcome following preventive intervention: a controlled study. In Ajemian I, Mount BM (eds): The RVH Manual on Palliative/Hospice Care. New York, Arno Press, 1980
9. Christie-Seely J: Terminal illness and death. In Christie-Seely J (ed): Working with the Family in Primary Care. New York, Praeger, 1984
10. Cramond WA: Psychotherapy of the dying patient. Br Med J 3:389, 1970

11. Duff RS, Hollingshead AB: Sickness and Society. New York, Harper & Row, 1968
12. Easson WM: Care of the young patient who is dying. JAMA 205:203, 1968
13. Engel GL: Grief and grieving. Am J Nurs 64:93, 1964
14. Fox R: Experiment Perilous. Glencoe Ill, The Free Press, 1959
15. Fulton R: Death and dying: some sociologic aspects of terminal care. Mod Med 40:74, 1972
16. Gerle B, Lunden G, Sandblom P: The patient with inoperable cancer from the psychiatric and social standpoints. Cancer 13:1206, 1960
17. Geyman JP: Dying and death of a family member. J Fam Pract 17:125, 1983
18. Gibson J, Derbyshire RC, Heffron WA, Roache C, Weihofen H: Right to die: a medical, moral, or legal decision. J Fam Pract 7:1047, 1978
19. Glaser BG, Strauss AL: Awareness of Dying. Chicago, Aldine, 1965
20. Goldin G: British hospices. In Bernstein E (ed): Medical and Health Annual. Chicago, Encyclopaedia Britannica, 1980
21. Hackett TP, Weisman AD: The treatment of dying. In Masserman JH (ed): Current Psychiatric Therapies, vol 2. New York, Grune & Stratton, 1962
22. Hackett TP, Weisman AD: Reactions to the imminence of death. In Grosser GH, Wechsler H, Greenblatt M (eds): The Threat of Impending Disaster. Cambridge, MIT Press, 1964
23. Helsing KJ, Syklo M: Mortality after bereavement. Am J Epidemiol 114:41, 1981
24. Hinton JM: The physical and mental distress of dying. QJ Med 32:1, 1963
25. Hinton J: Dying, 2nd ed. Harmondsworth, Penguin Books, 1972
26. Hinton J: Comparison of places and policies for terminal care. Lancet 1:29, 1979
27. Holland J: Psychological aspects of oncology. Med Clin North Am 61:737, 1977
28. Kastenbaum R: Death and dying. In Bernstein E (ed): Medical and Health Annual. Chicago, Encyclopaedia Britannica, 1979
29. Kelly OE, Murray WC: Make Today Count. New York, Delacorte, 1975
30. Kelly WP, Friesen S: Do cancer patients want to be told? Surgery 27:822, 1950
31. Krant MJ: The organized care of the dying patient. Hosp Pract 7:101, 1972
32. Kübler-Ross E: On Death and Dying. New York, Macmillan, 1969
33. Kübler-Ross E, Nighswonger CA: Death and American society. Transcript of a radio broadcast in the "Conversations at Chicago" series, produced by the University of Chicago, 1970
34. Lazare A: Unresolved grief. In Lazare A (ed): Outpatient Psychiatry: Diagnosis and Treatment. Baltimore, Williams & Wilkins, 1979
35. Litin EM: Should the cancer patient be told? Postgrad Med 28:470, 1960
36. May H, Breme FJ: SIDS family adjustment scale: A method of assessing family adjustment to sudden infant death syndrome. Omega 13:59, 1982
37. McCleave PB: Paradox: the physician and the clergyman. Marquette Med Rev 35:1, 1969
38. Mead M: The right to die. Nurs Outlook 16:20, 1968

39. Nighswonger CA: Ministry to the dying as a learning encounter. J Thanatol 1:101, 1971
40. Oken D: What to tell cancer patients. JAMA 175:1120, 1961
41. Parkes CM: Effects of bereavement on physical and mental health—a study of the medical records of widows. Br Med J 2:274, 1964
42. Parkes CM: Accuracy of predictions of survival in later stages of cancer. Br Med J 2:29, 1972
43. Parkes CM, Benjamin B, Fitzgerald RG: Broken heart: a statistical study of increased mortality among widowers. Br Med J 1:740, 1969
44. Payne EC: Depression and suicide. In Howells JG (ed): Modern Perspectives in the Psychiatry of Old Age. New York, Bruner/Mazel, 1975
45. Pemberton LB: Should we tell the truth? Resident Staff Physician 18:17, 1972
46. Pontoppidan H: Optimum care for hopelessly ill patients. N Engl J Med 295:362, 1976
47. Quint JC: Nurse and the Dying Patient. New York, Macmillan, 1967
48. Rabkin MT, Gillerman G, Rice NR: Orders not to resuscitate. N Engl J Med 295:364, 1976
49. Rakel RE: Principles of Family Medicine. Philadelphia, Saunders, 1977
50. Raphael B: Preventive intervention with the recently bereaved. Arch Gen Psychiatry 34:1450, 1977
51. Rees WD, Lutkins SG: Mortality of bereavement. Br Med J 4:13, 1967
52. Reich WT: The art of dying: dignity in death and life. New York Times, Jan 16, 1973
53. Saunders CM: The care of the dying. Gerontol Clin 9:385, 1967
54. Saunders CM: The care of the terminal stages of cancer. Ann R Col Surg Engl 41 (Suppl):162, 1967
55. Saunders C: Hospice care. Am J Med 65:726, 1978
56. Schleifer SJ, Keller SE, Camerino M, Thornton JC, Stein M: Suppression of lymphocyte stimulation following bereavement. JAMA 250:374, 1983
57. Shepard MW: This I believe . . . about questioning the right to die. Nurs Outlook 16:22, 1968
58. Stead EA Jr: If I become ill and unable to manage my own affairs. Resident Staff Physician 17:53, 1971
59. Thomas D: Collected Poems. New York, New Directions, 1957
60. Twycross R: The Relief of Pain: The Management of Terminal Disease. London, Edward Arnold Ltd, 1978
61. Vande Creek L: A homecare hospice profile: description, evaluation, and cost analysis. J Fam Pract 14:53, 1982
62. Vernick J, Karon M: Who's afraid of death on a leukemia ward? Am J Dis Child 109:393, 1965
63. Weisman AD: Misgivings and misconceptions in the psychiatric care of terminal patients. Psychiatry 33:67, 1970
64. Woodward KL, Gosnell M, Reese M, Coppola V, Liebert P: Living with dying. Newsweek, May 1, 1978
65. Wotton H: Upon the death of Sir Albert Morton's wife. In Hannah J (ed): The Poems of Sir Walter Raleigh with Those of Sir Henry Wotton. London, George Bell & Sons, 1892

# Index

Weins, A.N., 121
Weisman, A.D., 214, 215, 225, 226, 246, 247
Welch, C.E., 195
Westermeyer, J., 190, 196
Wexler, M., 51, 63
Whittemore, R., 47
"Why" questions, 99–100, 101
Williams, B., 196
Williams, J.G.L., 196
Winkelstein, C., 183, 196
Wittkower, E.D., 194
Wolberg, L.R., 70, 83

Wolf, S., 194
Woodward, K.L., 247
Workman, M.C., 196
Wotton, H., 235, 247
Wright, R.G., 196

**Z**

Zborowski, M., 199, 211
Zipes, D.P., 195
Zola, I.K., 199, 200–201, 211